Music Therapy for Dementia

Music Therapy for Dementia

A Dementia Care Essentials Guide

Peter M. Abraham, BSN, RN

Music Therapy for Dementia
A Dementia Care Essentials Guide

Contact Info: author@2abraham.com

First Edition: August 2024

DEDICATION

This book and the Dementia Care Essentials series it is part of are dedicated to multiple parties that helped shape my experiences and wisdom in caring for loved ones suffering from various types of dementia. I've worked with loved ones with dementia in long-term care as a registered nurse supervisor and as a hospice case manager. Caregivers and family members provided the most significant insights over the years.

Deborah, the wife of an Alzheimer's hospice at-home patient, provided insight into how the brains of dementia patients can be thought of like an electric clock. Most of the time, the clock is short-circuited and, therefore, not working correctly, but at times, as the clock's hands turn, the short-circuit goes away. For a fleeting time, a day or so, the person appears as if they don't have dementia.

Kathy is one of four daughters of a dementia patient for whom I provided care in a memory care center raised thought-provoking questions about the ethical dilemma of waking loved ones with dementia who want to sleep all the time to feed them vs. just letting them sleep.

Linda, who worked alongside me with a dementia patient, a former registered nurse herself, helped me understand other applications of validation therapy (a set of strategies and techniques that will be discussed in this book), such as rolling with resistance, which included accepting the nickname of "Jack," rather than my desire to be called Peter.

Jed, for whom I cared for his mother at home and then within a memory care center, reminded me of the actual cost that cannot be measured in terms of money of being a family caregiver.

Then there's our family journey, where my mother-in-law developed mixed dementia -- Alzheimer's disease plus vascular dementia – and was being cared for at home by her late husband, and then in a memory care center after he died suddenly.

More family members are involved, each helping me gain wisdom not taught in books. It is to all of these families and caregivers, as well as my late mother-in-law, Loris, and my wife, Laura, to whom this book and the others in this series are dedicated.

Table of Contents

Introduction

I know the journey you're on isn't an easy one. Caring for someone with dementia can be a challenging, often overwhelming experience. As an experienced nurse who's worked in long-term care and hospice, I've witnessed firsthand the daily struggles that families and caregivers face. I've seen the confusion in your loved one's eyes, the frustration in your voice, and the love that keeps you going despite it all.

Dementia is a unique beast. It's as if your loved one is moving forward in time physically, but mentally, emotionally, and functionally; they're journeying backward, gradually becoming more dependent - much like a newborn. And to complicate matters further, they might not even realize they have dementia. It's a situation that can leave even the most patient caregiver feeling lost and overwhelmed.

That's why I felt compelled to write this book. My goal is to offer you a beacon of hope in the form of music therapy - a powerful tool that can help manage behaviors and symptoms associated with dementia. But don't worry, the strategies we'll explore here aren't just limited to music; they'll benefit many aspects of your caregiving journey.

I've structured this book with you, the caregiver, at the forefront of my mind. We'll begin by discussing an often-overlooked but crucial aspect: self-care. When someone you love is battling a long-term illness like dementia - which can span decades - it affects the entire family. You, as a caregiver, are also experiencing your form of suffering, and we must address that.

From there, we'll delve into practical tips, including the importance of early legal and financial planning. It may not be the most exciting topic, but trust me, it's crucial for protecting both you and your loved one down the road.

We'll then explore validation therapy and other communication techniques. These skills will prove invaluable not just in dementia care, but in navigating all sorts of tricky situations life might throw your way.

The heart of our journey together will focus on integrating music therapy into dementia care. We'll explore how melodies can unlock memories, soothe agitation, and create moments of joy in even the most challenging times.

Lastly, recognizing that many individuals with dementia eventually require end-of-life care, we'll gently address this vital topic, providing you with the knowledge and emotional support to navigate this final stage with grace and compassion.

Remember, you're not alone on this journey. This book is more than just a guide - it's a companion, a source of support, and a reminder of the incredible difference you're making in your loved one's life. The road ahead may be challenging, but you can do this with the right tools, knowledge, and a sprinkle of music.

So, let's embark on this journey together, exploring the transformative power of music in dementia care. I hope that by the time you finish this book, you'll have new strategies to implement and a renewed sense of hope and purpose in your caregiving role.

Are you ready? Let's begin.

Caring for the Caregiver

Caring for a loved one with dementia is a journey of profound love and dedication, but it's also one of the most challenging roles a person can undertake. As caregivers and family members, you stand at the forefront of this complex and often overwhelming experience. Your commitment to providing compassionate care is admirable, yet it's crucial to recognize the significant impact this role can have on your well-being.

The Emotional and Physical Toll

The path of a dementia caregiver is paved with a myriad of emotions and physical demands that can test even the strongest individuals. Let's explore the multifaceted nature of this toll:

Emotional Challenges:

1. Grief and loss: Watching a loved one's cognitive decline
2. Guilt: Feeling inadequate or struggling with difficult decisions
3. Anxiety: Worrying about the future and managing daily uncertainties
4. Frustration: Dealing with repetitive behaviors and communication barriers
5. Isolation: Experiencing a shrinking social circle and loss of personal time

Physical Demands:

- Sleep deprivation due to irregular sleep patterns of the care recipient
- Chronic stress leading to weakened immune function
- Neglect of personal health needs and medical appointments
- Physical strain from assisting with mobility and personal care tasks
- Exhaustion from constant vigilance and round-the-clock care

These emotional and physical challenges create a complex web that can entangle even the most resilient caregivers. It's essential to recognize that experiencing these difficulties doesn't reflect on your capabilities or dedication – it's a natural response to an extraordinarily demanding situation.

Common Caregiver Emotions	Physical Manifestations	Potential Long-term Consequences
Sadness, Grief	Fatigue, Weakened Immunity	Depression, Chronic Illness
Anxiety, Worry	Insomnia, Muscle Tension	Anxiety Disorders, Chronic Pain
Frustration, Anger	High Blood Pressure, Headaches	Cardiovascular Issues, Migraines
Guilt, Self-doubt	Appetite Changes, Digestive Issues	Eating Disorders, Gastrointestinal Problems

Recognizing the Signs of Caregiver Burnout

Caregiver burnout is a state of physical, emotional, and mental exhaustion that can creep up slowly or suddenly. Awareness of the warning signs is crucial to prevent reaching this critical point. Here are key indicators to watch for:

1. **Emotional Signs:**
    - Feeling overwhelmed or constantly worried
    - Experiencing mood swings or irritability
    - Losing interest in activities once enjoyed
    - Feeling hopeless, helpless, or alone

2. **Physical Signs:**
    - Frequently falling ill or feeling constantly tired
    - Changes in appetite or sleep patterns
    - Neglecting personal hygiene or appearance
    - Developing new health problems or exacerbating existing ones
3. **Behavioral Signs:**
    - Withdrawing from friends and family
    - Procrastinating on important tasks
    - Using alcohol, food, or medications to cope
    - Lashing out at the person with dementia or others
4. **Cognitive Signs:**
    - Difficulty concentrating or making decisions
    - Forgetfulness in daily tasks
    - Trouble problem-solving or thinking clearly
    - Negative thought patterns or constant worry

Self-Assessment Checklist for Caregiver Burnout:

Warning Sign	Frequency (Rarely/Sometimes/Often/Always)
I feel exhausted even after sleeping.	
I catch myself yelling or arguing more often.	
I've stopped seeing friends or engaging in hobbies.	
I feel resentful towards the person I'm caring for.	
I worry constantly about the future.	
I neglect my own health needs.	
I have trouble falling asleep or staying asleep.	
I feel like I can't do anything right.	

If you find yourself answering "Often" or "Always" to several of these statements, it may be time to seek additional support and focus on self-care strategies.

Remember, recognizing these signs is not an admission of failure but a crucial step in maintaining your ability to provide care. By acknowledging the challenges and being vigilant about your well-being, you can take proactive steps to prevent burnout and ensure that you can continue to provide the best possible care for your loved one with dementia. Your role is invaluable, and by taking care of yourself, you're also ensuring the best care for your loved one.

Understanding the Importance of Self-Care

As caregivers and family members supporting individuals with dementia, you're intimately familiar with the concept of care. However, it's crucial to remember that care must also extend to you. Self-care isn't a luxury; it's a necessity that directly impacts your ability to provide compassionate, practical support to your loved ones or patients.

The Impact of Self-Care on Caregiving Quality

The quality of care you provide is intrinsically linked to your well-being. When you prioritize self-care, you benefit yourself and enhance your capacity to care for others. Let's explore how self-care positively influences various aspects of caregiving:

1. **Enhanced Emotional Resilience**
    - Better equipped to handle stress and emotional challenges
    - Increased patience and empathy in difficult situations
    - Improved ability to maintain a calm demeanor
2. **Improved Physical Stamina**
    - Greater energy to perform caregiving tasks
    - Reduced risk of caregiver-related injuries
    - Increased overall health, leading to fewer sick days
3. **Sharpened Mental Acuity**
    - Better decision-making skills in critical situations
    - Improved memory and attention to detail
    - Enhanced problem-solving abilities
4. **Strengthened Relationships**
    - more positive interactions with the care recipient

- Healthier boundaries with family members and healthcare professionals
- Improved communication skills

5. **Increased Caregiving Longevity**
    - Reduced risk of burnout and compassion fatigue
    - Sustained ability to provide care over extended periods
    - Greater job satisfaction for professional caregivers

Self-Care Practice	Benefits to Caregiver	Impact on Caregiving Quality
Regular Exercise	Improved physical health, stress relief	Increased energy, better mood during care
Adequate Sleep	Better cognitive function, emotional stability	Enhanced decision-making, patience in care
Mindfulness/Meditation	Reduced anxiety, improved focus	Increased presence and empathy in interactions
Social Connections	Emotional support, reduced isolation	Renewed energy and perspective in caregiving

Overcoming Guilt and Prioritizing Personal Needs

One of the most significant barriers to self-care for caregivers is the pervasive feeling of guilt. It's common to feel that taking time for yourself is selfish or detracts from the care you should provide. However, overcoming this guilt is essential for sustainable caregiving. Here's how to reframe your thinking and prioritize your needs:

Understanding Guilt in Caregiving:

- Recognize that guilt is a common and normal emotion for caregivers
- Acknowledge that guilt often stems from unrealistic expectations of yourself
- Realize that neglecting your needs can lead to resentment and diminished care quality

Strategies for Overcoming Caregiver Guilt:

1. **Reframe Your Perspective**
    - View self-care as a necessary part of providing good care
    - Understand that taking care of yourself allows you to be more present and effective
    - Recognize that you're modeling healthy behavior for others
2. **Set Realistic Expectations**
    - Accept that you can't do everything perfectly
    - Understand that it's okay to have limits and boundaries
    - Recognize that asking for help is a sign of strength, not weakness
3. **Practice Self-Compassion**
    - Treat yourself with the same kindness you show to others
    - Acknowledge your efforts and successes, no matter how small
    - Use positive self-talk to counter guilty thoughts

4. **Educate Yourself and Others**
    - Learn about the importance of self-care in caregiving literature
    - Share information with family members to gain their support
    - Discuss the benefits of caregiver well-being with healthcare professionals
5. **Start Small and Build**
    - Begin with short periods of self-care to ease into the practice
    - Gradually increase the time and frequency of self-care activities
    - Celebrate each step you take towards prioritizing your needs

Practical Steps to Prioritize Personal Needs:

- **Schedule Self-Care**: Block out time in your calendar for activities that rejuvenate you
- **Create a Self-Care Plan**: Develop a written plan outlining your self-care goals and strategies
- **Communicate Your Needs**: Clearly express your needs to family members and support networks
- **Use Respite Care**: Take advantage of respite services to get regular breaks
- **Join Support Groups**: Connect with other caregivers who understand your challenges
- **Seek Professional Help**: Consider therapy or counseling to work through feelings of guilt

Common Guilt-Inducing Thoughts	Reframed Perspective
"I should be doing more."	"I'm doing my best, and that's enough."
"Taking a break is selfish."	"Taking care of myself helps me provide better care."
"Nobody else can care for them like I can."	"Accepting help allows for fresh energy in caregiving."
"I don't deserve to enjoy myself."	"My well-being is important and valid."

Remember, prioritizing your needs isn't selfish—it's essential. You can continue providing the high-quality, compassionate care that your loved ones or patients deserve by taking care of yourself. Self-care is integral to the caregiving journey, benefiting you and those you care for. Embrace it without guilt, knowing that you're making a wise investment in your ability to care for others.

Physical Self-Care Strategies

Your physical health is the foundation of your ability to provide care as a caregiver. While putting your needs last is easy, maintaining your physical well-being is crucial for you and your loved one. Let's explore practical strategies to keep your body healthy and energized.

Maintaining a Healthy Diet

A nutritious diet is essential for sustaining your energy levels and overall health. Here are some strategies to ensure you're fueling your body properly:

1. **Plan and Prepare Meals in Advance**
    - Use weekends or less busy times to batch-cook meals
    - Freeze portions for easy reheating during hectic days
    - Prepare healthy snacks to avoid reaching for processed foods
2. **Focus on Nutrient-Dense Foods**

- Incorporate a variety of colorful fruits and vegetables
- Choose whole grains over refined carbohydrates
- Include lean proteins like fish, poultry, beans, and nuts
- Don't forget healthy fats from sources like avocados and olive oil

3. **Stay Hydrated**
    - Keep a water bottle with you throughout the day
    - Set reminders to drink water regularly
    - Include hydrating foods like cucumbers and watermelon in your diet
4. **Mindful Eating**
    - Take time to sit down and enjoy your meals
    - Avoid eating while multitasking or when stressed
    - Listen to your body's hunger and fullness cues
5. **Seek Support**
    - Ask family members or friends to help with meal preparation
    - Consider meal delivery services for fresh, healthy options
    - Consult a nutritionist for personalized dietary advice if needed

Meal Type	Quick and Healthy Options
Breakfast	Greek yogurt with berries and nuts, overnight oats, whole grain toast with avocado.
Lunch	Mixed green salad with grilled chicken, whole grain wrap with hummus and vegetables.
Dinner	Baked salmon with roasted vegetables, vegetarian chili, stir-fry with tofu and mixed veggies.
Snacks	Apple slices with almond butter, carrot sticks with hummus, and a handful of mixed nuts.

Incorporating Regular Exercise

Exercise is not just about physical fitness; it's a powerful stress reliever and mood booster. Here's how to make physical activity a regular part of your routine:

1. **Find Activities You Enjoy**
    - Experiment with different types of exercise to find what you like
    - Consider activities that can involve your loved one, like gentle walks
    - Try yoga or tai chi for both physical and mental benefits
2. **Set Realistic Goals**
    - Start small. Even 10 minutes a day can make a difference
    - Gradually increase duration and intensity as you build stamina
    - Celebrate your progress, no matter how small

3. **Make It Convenient**
    - Keep exercise equipment at home for quick workouts
    - Use online fitness videos for guided sessions
    - Take advantage of small pockets of time throughout the day
4. **Incorporate Movement into Daily Tasks**
    - Do calf raises while washing dishes
    - Perform stretches during TV commercials
    - Take the stairs instead of the elevator when possible
5. **Seek Support and Accountability**
    - Join a caregiver fitness group or online community
    - Use fitness apps to track your progress
    - Ask a friend or family member to be your exercise buddy

Exercise Type	Benefits	Caregiver-Friendly Examples
Cardiovascular	Improves heart health, boosts energy	Brisk walking, dancing, stationary cycling
Strength Training	Builds muscle, supports bone health	Bodyweight exercises, resistance bands, light dumbbells
Flexibility	Reduces muscle tension, improves mobility	Gentle stretching, yoga, tai chi
Balance	Prevents falls, improves stability	Single-leg stands, heel-to-toe walk, balance board

Ensuring Adequate Sleep and Rest

Quality sleep is crucial for your physical and mental well-being. Here are strategies to improve your sleep habits:

1. **Establish a Consistent Sleep Schedule**
    - Try to go to bed and wake up at the same time each day
    - Create a relaxing bedtime routine to signal your body it's time to sleep
    - Avoid screens for at least an hour before bedtime
2. **Optimize Your Sleep Environment**
    - Keep your bedroom cool, dark, and quiet
    - Invest in a comfortable mattress and pillows
    - Use white noise or earplugs if needed to block out disturbances
3. **Manage Nighttime Caregiving**
    - Use night lights to avoid fully waking up for nighttime checks
    - Consider assistive devices like bed alarms to alert you when needed
    - Take turns with other family members for nighttime care if possible
4. **Practice Relaxation Techniques**
    - Try deep breathing exercises before bed
    - Use guided imagery or meditation to calm your mind
    - Practice progressive muscle relaxation to release physical tension

5. **Be Mindful of Diet and Exercise**
    - Avoid caffeine and heavy meals close to bedtime
    - Exercise regularly, but not too close to bedtime
    - Limit alcohol, as it can disrupt sleep patterns
6. **Prioritize Rest During the Day**
    - Take short power naps (15-20 minutes) when possible
    - Use respite care to get a whole night's sleep occasionally
    - Practice mindfulness or meditation for mental rest during the day

Sleep Challenge	Potential Solution
Difficulty falling asleep	Practice a calming bedtime routine, and try relaxation techniques.
Waking up during the night	Keep a notepad by your bed to jot down thoughts, and use white noise.
Early morning wakings	Ensure your room is dark, and consider adjusting your sleep schedule.
Feeling unrested after sleep	Evaluate your sleep environment and consult a doctor about sleep quality.

Remember, taking care of your physical health is not selfish—it's a necessary part of being an effective caregiver. By prioritizing your diet, exercise, and sleep, you're ensuring you have the strength and energy to provide the best care possible for your loved one. Start with small, manageable changes, and be patient with yourself as you develop these healthy habits. Your body—and your loved one—will thank you for it.

Emotional and Mental Well-being

As a caregiver, tending to your emotional and mental health is just as crucial as maintaining your physical well-being. The demands of caring for a loved one can significantly toll your psychological state, making it essential to develop strategies that nurture your inner self. Let's explore some effective methods to support your emotional and mental well-being.

Practicing Mindfulness and Meditation

Mindfulness and meditation are powerful tools for managing stress, improving focus, and cultivating inner peace. These practices can be particularly beneficial for caregivers, offering moments of calm in challenging situations.

Benefits of Mindfulness and Meditation for Caregivers:

- Reduced stress and anxiety
- Improved emotional regulation
- Enhanced ability to focus and concentrate
- Increased self-awareness and empathy
- Better sleep quality
- Boosted immune function

How to Incorporate Mindfulness and Meditation into Your Daily Routine:

1. **Start Small**
    - Begin with just 5 minutes a day
    - Gradually increase the duration as you become more comfortable
2. **Choose a Consistent Time and Place**
    - Set aside a specific time each day for your practice
    - Create a quiet, comfortable space for meditation

3. **Explore Different Techniques**
    - Try guided meditations using apps or online resources
    - Experiment with breathing exercises, body scans, or loving-kindness meditation
    - Practice mindful activities like walking or eating
4. **Be Patient and Non-Judgmental**
    - Remember that it's normal for your mind to wander
    - Gently bring your attention back to your focus point without self-criticism
5. **Integrate Mindfulness into Daily Activities**
    - Practice being fully present during routine tasks like washing dishes or folding laundry
    - Take mindful breaks throughout the day, even if just for a few deep breaths

Mindfulness Technique	Description	When to Use
Breath Awareness	Focus on the sensation of breathing, noticing each inhale and exhale	Any time, especially during stressful moments
Body Scan	Systematically relax each part of your body from head to toe	Before bed or during breaks
Loving-Kindness Meditation	Direct positive thoughts and wishes towards yourself and others	When feeling overwhelmed or frustrated
Mindful Walking	Pay attention to each step and your surroundings while walking	During outdoor breaks or while moving between tasks

Journaling and Emotional Expression

Journaling is a powerful tool for processing emotions, gaining clarity, and fostering self-reflection. For caregivers, it can serve as a private outlet for expressing the complex feelings often accompanying caregiving.

Benefits of Journaling for Caregivers:

- Emotional release and stress reduction
- Increased self-awareness and problem-solving
- Documentation of caregiving journey and memories
- Opportunity for a gratitude practice
- Improved communication skills

Tips for Effective Journaling:

1. **Choose Your Medium**
   - Traditional pen and paper
   - Digital journaling apps or word processors
   - Audio recordings or voice memos
2. **Set Aside Regular Time**
   - Aim for consistency, even if it's just a few minutes daily
   - Choose a time when you're least likely to be interrupted
3. **Write Freely Without Judgment**
   - Don't worry about grammar, spelling, or structure
   - Let your thoughts flow without censoring yourself

4. **Use Prompts When Needed**
    - "Today, I felt..."
    - "I'm grateful for..."
    - "A challenge I faced today was..."
    - "Something I learned about myself is..."
5. **Reflect on Your Entries**
    - Periodically review your journal to observe patterns and growth
    - Use insights gained to inform your self-care and caregiving strategies
6. **Explore Different Journaling Techniques**
    - Gratitude journaling
    - Stream of consciousness writing
    - Dialogue journaling (writing conversations with yourself or others)
    - Art journaling (combining writing with visual elements)

Journaling Method	Description	Benefit for Caregivers
Gratitude Journal	Daily list of things you're thankful for	Shifts focus to positive aspects of caregiving
Emotional Release Writing	Unfiltered expression of feelings and thoughts	Helps process difficult emotions and experiences
Problem-Solving Journal	Writing out challenges and brainstorming solutions	Enhances coping skills and decision-making
Reflection Journal	Regular entries about personal growth and insights	Promotes self-awareness and resilience

Seeking Professional Mental Health Support

While self-care practices are essential, there may be times when professional support is necessary. Seeking help from a mental health professional is a sign of strength and can provide valuable tools for managing the emotional challenges of caregiving.

Signs You May Benefit from Professional Support:

- Persistent feelings of sadness, anxiety, or hopelessness
- Difficulty managing anger or frustration
- Feeling overwhelmed or unable to cope
- Changes in sleep patterns or appetite
- Loss of interest in activities you once enjoyed
- Thoughts of self-harm or suicide

Types of Professional Mental Health Support:

1. **Individual Therapy**
    - One-on-one sessions with a licensed therapist or counselor.
    - Can focus on specific caregiving challenges or broader emotional issues.
2. **Support Groups**
    - Facilitated groups for caregivers to share experiences and coping strategies.
    - It can be in-person or online.
3. **Cognitive Behavioral Therapy (CBT)**
    - It helps identify and change negative thought patterns and behaviors.
    - It is particularly effective for managing anxiety and depression.

4. **Mindfulness-Based Stress Reduction (MBSR)**
   - Combines mindfulness meditation and yoga to reduce stress.
   - Often offered in 8-week programs.
5. **Telehealth Options**
   - Virtual therapy sessions via video call or phone.
   - Convenient for caregivers with limited time or transportation.

Steps to Access Mental Health Support:

1. **Consult Your Primary Care Physician**
   - Discuss your concerns and get referrals to mental health professionals.
2. **Check with Your Insurance Provider**
   - Understand your coverage for mental health services.
   - Get a list of in-network providers.
3. **Research Local Resources**
   - Contact local hospitals or community centers for caregiver support programs.
   - Look into non-profit organizations specializing in your loved one's condition.
4. **Consider Online Platforms**
   - Explore reputable online therapy services.
   - Look for platforms that offer specific support for caregivers.

5. **Don't Hesitate to Try Different Options**
    - Switching therapists is okay if you don't feel a good connection.
    - Explore different types of therapy to find what works best for you.

Type of Support	Best For	Potential Drawbacks
Individual Therapy	Personalized attention, deep exploration of issues	It can be costly, time-consuming
Support Groups	Shared experiences, practical advice from peers	Less individual focus and may not address specific needs
Online Therapy	Convenience, flexibility in scheduling	Potential technology issues, less personal connection
Crisis Hotlines	Immediate support during acute stress or emergencies	Not suitable for ongoing, in-depth support

Remember, taking care of your emotional and mental well-being is not a luxury—it's a necessity. By practicing mindfulness, journaling, and seeking professional support when needed, you're investing in your ability to provide compassionate care. Be patient with yourself as you explore these strategies, and remember that it's okay to prioritize your mental health. A mentally healthy caregiver is better equipped to face the challenges of caregiving with resilience and grace.

Building a Support Network

As a caregiver, it's crucial to remember that you don't have to face this journey alone. Building a solid support network can provide emotional support, practical assistance, and valuable resources. Let's explore how you can create and nurture a network that will sustain you through the challenges of caregiving.

Joining Caregiver Support Groups

Caregiver support groups offer a unique opportunity to connect with others who truly understand your experiences. These groups can be invaluable sources of emotional support, practical advice, and camaraderie.

Benefits of Joining Caregiver Support Groups:

- Emotional validation and understanding
- Sharing of practical tips and resources
- Reduced feelings of isolation and loneliness
- Opportunity to help others and feel empowered
- Access to educational resources and expert speakers

Types of Caregiver Support Groups:

1. **In-Person Groups**
    - Often held at community centers, hospitals, or religious organizations
    - Provide face-to-face interaction and immediate support
2. **Online Forums and Groups**
    - Accessible from anywhere, at any time
    - Offer anonymity and convenience
3. **Condition-Specific Groups**
    - Focus on caregivers dealing with particular illnesses or conditions
    - Provide specialized information and understanding
4. **Demographic-Specific Groups**
    - Cater to specific caregiver demographics (e.g., spouses, adult children, young caregivers)
    - Address unique challenges faced by different caregiver populations

How to Find and Join a Support Group:

1. Research local options through hospitals, community centers, or disease-specific organizations
2. Explore online platforms like Facebook groups or caregiver-specific websites
3. Ask your healthcare provider for recommendations
4. Consider starting your group if you can't find one that meets your needs

Type of Group	Pros	Cons
In-Person	Personal connection, immediate support	Time commitment, transportation needed
Online	Convenient, accessible 24/7	Lack of face-to-face interaction
Condition-Specific	Targeted advice, shared experiences	It may be limited in availability
General Caregiver	Broader perspective, diverse experiences	May lack specificity for your situation

Involving Family and Friends

Your existing network of family and friends can be a powerful source of support. However, many caregivers struggle with asking for help or feel guilty about burdening others. Remember, most people want to help but may not know how.

Strategies for Involving Family and Friends:

1. **Be Specific About Your Needs**
    - Create a list of tasks that others can help with
    - Be clear about what kind of support you're looking for (practical, emotional, etc.)

2. **Use Technology to Coordinate**
    - Utilize care coordination apps or shared calendars
    - Set up a group chat or email thread for updates and requests
3. **Educate Them About Your Caregiving Situation**
    - Share information about your loved one's condition
    - Help them understand the challenges you face
4. **Foster Ongoing Connections**
    - Schedule regular check-ins or social gatherings
    - Encourage friends and family to maintain a relationship with your care recipient
5. **Express Gratitude**
    - Thank helpers for their support, no matter how small
    - Let them know the positive impact of their assistance

Overcoming Barriers to Asking for Help:

- Recognize that accepting help benefits both you and your care recipient
- Start small if you're uncomfortable asking for big favors
- Remember that people often want to help but don't know how

Practice asking for help to become more comfortable with it Type of Support	Examples	How to Ask
Practical Assistance	Meal preparation, house cleaning, errands	"Could you pick up groceries for us this week?"
Respite Care	Sitting with the care recipient, overnight care	"Can you stay with Mom for a few hours on Saturday?"
Emotional Support	Listening, checking in, offering encouragement	"I'm having a tough week. Could we chat over coffee?"
Financial Help	Assistance with bills, fundraising	"We're struggling with medical expenses. Can you help us set up a fundraiser?"

Utilizing Community Resources and Respite Care

Community resources and respite care services can provide crucial support, allowing you to take breaks and access specialized assistance. These resources can help prevent burnout and ensure better care for you and your loved one.

Types of Community Resources:

1. **Area Agencies on Aging (AAA)**
   - Provide information, referrals, and sometimes direct services
   - Often offer caregiver support programs and resources

2. **Local Senior Centers**
    - May offer adult daycare programs
    - Provide social activities and meals for seniors
3. **Faith-Based Organizations**
    - Often have volunteer programs to assist caregivers
    - May offer support groups or counseling services
4. **Non-Profit Organizations**
    - Condition-specific organizations often have local chapters with resources
    - May offer educational workshops, support groups, or financial assistance

Respite Care Options:

1. **In-Home Respite**
    - Professional caregivers come to your home
    - Can range from a few hours to overnight care
2. **Adult Day Centers**
    - Provide care and activities during daytime hours
    - Often include meals and social interaction for care recipients
3. **Residential Respite**
    - Short-term stays at assisted living facilities or nursing homes
    - Allows for extended breaks or travel
4. **Volunteer Respite Programs**
    - Often run by community organizations or faith groups
    - May offer limited hours of free care

Steps to Access Community Resources and Respite Care:

1. Contact your local AAA for a comprehensive list of resources
2. Speak with your loved one's healthcare provider for recommendations
3. Research condition-specific organizations for specialized support
4. Explore online directories of senior services and respite care options
5. Consult with a social worker or case manager for personalized guidance

Resource Type	Services Offered	How to Access
Area Agency on Aging	Information, referrals, caregiver support programs	Call the local office or visit the website
Adult Day Centers	Daytime care, activities, meals	Contact the center directly for a tour and assessment
Home Health Agencies	In-home care, nursing services, respite	Get a referral from a doctor or contact an agency
Volunteer Programs	Companionship, errands, light housekeeping	Contact local senior centers or faith organizations

Remember, building a strong support network is an ongoing process. Finding the right combination of support groups, family involvement, and community resources that work for you may take time. Be patient with yourself and persistent in seeking out the help you need. By creating a robust support system, you're taking care of yourself and ensuring you can provide the best possible care for your loved one.

Don't hesitate to reach out and accept help when it's offered. Your role as a caregiver is invaluable, and by taking care of yourself through building a strong support network, you're ensuring that you can continue to provide compassionate care for the long term.

Time Management and Organization

As a caregiver, you often juggle multiple responsibilities, making time management and organization crucial skills. Effective planning can help reduce stress, increase efficiency, and ensure you and your loved one receive the care and attention needed. Let's explore strategies to help you manage your time and effectively organize your caregiving duties.

Creating a Caregiving Schedule

A well-structured caregiving schedule can provide a sense of routine and predictability, which benefits both you and your care recipient. Here's how to create an effective caregiving schedule:

1. **Assess Care Needs**
   - List all daily, weekly, and monthly tasks required for your loved one's care.
   - Include medical appointments, medication times, and personal care routines.
2. **Prioritize Tasks**
   - Identify critical tasks that must be done at specific times.
   - Determine which tasks are flexible and can be rescheduled if needed.
3. **Create a Template**
   - Use a digital calendar or a large paper calendar.
   - Color-code different types of activities for easy visualization.
4. **Include Self-Care**
   - Schedule time for your appointments, breaks, and activities.
   - Block out time for sleep and regular meals.

5. **Be Realistic**
    - Allow extra time for tasks, as caregiving often takes longer than expected.
    - Build buffer time for unexpected events or emergencies.
6. **Review and Adjust Regularly**
    - Reassess the schedule weekly or monthly.
    - Make changes as care needs evolve or your situation changes.

Time	Task	Responsible Person
7:00 AM	Morning medications and breakfast	Primary Caregiver
9:00 AM	Personal care and dressing	Home Health Aide
11:00 AM	Physical therapy exercises	Primary Caregiver
1:00 PM	Lunch and afternoon medications	Family Member
3:00 PM	Social activity or rest	Volunteer Companion
6:00 PM	Dinner and evening medications	Primary Caregiver
8:00 PM	Bedtime routine	Primary Caregiver

Delegating Tasks and Accepting Help

Delegating tasks and accepting help are essential for maintaining your well-being and ensuring comprehensive care for your loved one. Here's how to approach delegation effectively:

1. **Identify Delegable Tasks**
    - Make a list of tasks that don't require your specific expertise.
    - Consider which tasks others might enjoy or be well-suited to perform.

2. **Match Tasks to Helpers**
    - Consider the skills, availability, and preferences of potential helpers.
    - Assign tasks that align with each person's strengths and schedules.
3. **Communicate Clearly**
    - Provide detailed instructions for each task.
    - Set clear expectations for how and when tasks should be completed.
4. **Express Appreciation**
    - Thank helpers for their contributions, no matter how small.
    - Acknowledge the positive impact of their assistance.
5. **Be Open to Different Methods**
    - Recognize that others may complete tasks differently than you would.
    - Focus on results rather than specific methods when possible.
6. **Overcome Reluctance to Delegate**
    - Remind yourself that accepting help benefits both you and your loved one.
    - Start small if you're uncomfortable with extensive delegation.

Strategies for Effective Delegation:

- Use a shared task list or care coordination app.
- Rotate responsibilities among family members.
- Consider hiring professional help for specialized tasks.
- Utilize volunteer services for non-medical assistance.

Task Category	Examples	Potential Delegates
Household Chores	Cleaning, laundry, yard work	Family members, hired help, volunteers
Errands	Grocery shopping, pharmacy runs	Friends, neighbors, delivery services
Personal Care	Bathing, dressing, grooming	Home health aides, trained family members
Social Support	Companionship, activities	Friends, volunteers, adult day programs
Medical Management	Medication reminders, doctor appointments	Nursing services, tech solutions, family members

Using Technology to Streamline Caregiving Duties

Technology can be a powerful ally in managing caregiving responsibilities. Various tools can help simplify your caregiving journey, from organizing tasks to monitoring health. Here's how to leverage technology effectively:

1. **Care Coordination Apps**
   - Use apps designed for caregivers to manage schedules, tasks, and communication.
   - Examples: Caring Village, Lotsa Helping Hands, and CaringBridge.
2. **Medication Management Tools**
   - Utilize apps or smart pill dispensers to track and remind about medications.
   - Consider: Medisafe, PillPack, and Hero.

3. **Health Monitoring Devices**
    - Implement wearable devices or smart home sensors for health tracking.
    - Options: Fall detection devices, blood pressure monitors, GPS trackers.
4. **Communication Tools**
    - Use video calling apps to connect with your loved one and other caregivers.
    - Try: Skype, FaceTime, or Zoom.
5. **Online Support and Education**
    - Access online forums, webinars, and caregiver support and education courses.
    - Explore: Family Caregiver Alliance, AARP Caregiver Resource Center.
6. **Smart Home Devices**
    - Implement voice-activated assistants and smart home technology for added convenience and safety.
    - Consider: Amazon Alexa, Google Home, smart thermostats, and automated lighting.

Tips for Implementing Caregiving Technology:

- Start with one or two tools and gradually add more as needed.
- Ensure all caregivers are trained on how to use the technology.
- Regularly review and update your tech tools as care needs change.
- Consider the comfort level of your care recipient with technology.

Technology Type	Benefits	Considerations
Care Coordination Apps	Improved communication, task management	Requires all caregivers to adopt and use consistently
Health Monitoring Devices	Early detection of health issues, increased independence	It may require professional setup, ongoing costs
Medication Management Tools	Reduced medication errors, improved adherence	Need for regular updates, potential tech glitches
Smart Home Devices	Enhanced safety, convenience for daily tasks	Initial setup cost, learning curve for usage

Remember, effective time management and organization are ongoing processes. Be patient with yourself as you implement these strategies, and don't hesitate to adjust your approach as needed. You can create a more manageable and sustainable caregiving routine by creating a structured schedule, delegating tasks, and leveraging technology.

These tools and strategies are meant to support you, not add stress. Please choose the best methods for your unique situation and gradually incorporate them into your caregiving routine. With time and practice, you'll likely find that improved organization leads to more quality time with your loved one and better self-care for you as a caregiver.

Maintaining Personal Identity and Interests

As a caregiver, it's easy to become so immersed in your responsibilities that you lose sight of your identity and interests. However, maintaining a sense of self is crucial for your well-being and can make you a more effective caregiver. Let's explore ways to nurture your identity and interests while balancing your caregiving duties.

Pursuing Hobbies and Passions

Engaging in activities you enjoy is not a luxury—it's necessary to maintain your mental and emotional health. Here's how to keep your hobbies and passions alive:

1. **Identify Time Pockets**
    - Look for small windows of time in your schedule
    - Consider early mornings, during care recipient's naps, or after bedtime
2. **Adapt Your Hobbies**
    - Find ways to engage in your interests in shorter time frames
    - Look for portable versions of your hobbies
3. **Involve Your Care Recipient**
    - When possible, find ways to include your loved one in your activities
    - This can provide stimulation for them and enjoyment for you both
4. **Use Technology**
    - Explore online classes or virtual communities related to your interests
    - Use apps or online resources to engage in hobbies remotely
5. **Schedule Regular "Me Time"**
    - Block out time in your calendar for your interests
    - Treat this time as crucial as any other appointment

Ideas for Maintaining Hobbies:

- Reading: Join an online book club or use audiobooks during commutes
- Art: Keep a sketchbook for quick drawing sessions
- Music: Create playlists to enjoy while performing caregiving tasks
- Gardening: Start a small indoor herb garden or tend to potted plants
- Exercise: Try short workout videos or practice yoga during breaks

Hobby Type	Adaptation for Caregivers	Benefits
Reading	E-books, audiobooks, short stories	Mental stimulation, stress relief
Crafting	Portable projects (knitting, sketching)	Creativity outlet, sense of accomplishment
Fitness	Short home workouts, walking	Physical health, energy boost
Cooking	Quick recipes, meal prep	Nutrition, enjoyment, potential involvement of care recipient

Staying Connected with Friends

Maintaining social connections is vital for your emotional well-being and provides a support system outside your caregiving role. Here are strategies to stay connected:

1. **Leverage Technology**
    - Use video calls, social media, or messaging apps to stay in touch
    - Join online groups or forums related to your interests

2. **Schedule Regular Check-ins**
    - Set up recurring phone calls or virtual coffee dates with friends
    - Use calendar reminders to prompt you to reach out
3. **Be Honest About Your Situation**
    - Share your caregiving challenges with trusted friends
    - Let them know how they can support you
4. **Plan for Social Activities**
    - Arrange respite care to allow for occasional outings
    - Invite friends for short visits at home when possible
5. **Involve Friends in Caregiving**
    - Ask friends to visit or spend time with your care recipient
    - This can provide you with a break while maintaining connections

Tips for Maintaining Friendships:

- Quality over quantity: Focus on nurturing a few close relationships
- Be present: When you do have time with friends, try to be fully engaged
- Share your caregiving journey: Allow friends to understand your life
- Accept help: Let friends support you in practical ways if they offer

Connection Type	Ideas for Caregivers	Potential Challenges
Virtual Meetups	Video chat coffee dates, online game nights	Technology issues, scheduling conflicts
In-Person Visits	Short home visits, park meetups	Limited time, need for care coverage
Group Activities	Book clubs, virtual workout groups	Finding common interests, time commitment
Caregiving Involvement	Friend visits with care recipient, help with tasks	Friends' comfort level with caregiving situation

Setting Personal Goals Outside of Caregiving

Setting and working towards personal goals can provide a sense of purpose and achievement beyond your caregiving role. Here's how to approach goal-setting:

1. **Reflect on Your Aspirations**
    - Think about what you want to achieve for yourself
    - Consider short-term and long-term goals
2. **Start Small**
    - Set realistic, achievable goals given your current situation
    - Break larger goals into smaller, manageable steps
3. **Make Goals SMART**
    - Specific, Measurable, Achievable, Relevant, Time-bound
    - This framework helps create clear, actionable goals

4. **Write Down Your Goals**
    - Use a journal or goal-tracking app to document your objectives
    - Regularly review and update your goals
5. **Seek Support**
    - Share your goals with friends or family who can encourage you
    - Consider finding an accountability partner
6. **Celebrate Progress**
    - Acknowledge and celebrate each step towards your goals
    - Use achievements as motivation to continue pursuing your aspirations

Examples of Personal Goals for Caregivers:

- Learning: Take an online course or learn a new language
- Health: Establish a regular exercise routine or improve eating habits
- Career: Maintain professional skills or explore part-time work options
- Creative: Start a blog, write a book, or create art
- Personal Growth: Practice mindfulness or develop a new skill

Goal Category	Example Goal	Potential Steps
Education	Complete an online certificate program	Research programs, allocate study time, set completion date
Health and Wellness	Establish a regular meditation practice.	Download the app, start with 5 minutes daily, and gradually increase the time.
Personal Development	Improve time management skills.	Read productivity books, try a time-blocking technique, and use organization apps.
Creative Expression	Write and publish a short story	Set writing schedule, join writing group, research publishing options

Remember, maintaining your identity and interests is not selfish—it's essential for your well-being and can make you a more effective and compassionate caregiver. By pursuing your hobbies, staying connected with friends, and setting personal goals, you're taking care of yourself and bringing fresh energy and perspective to your caregiving role.

Feeling guilty about taking time for yourself is normal, but remember that self-care is crucial to sustainable caregiving—your loved one benefits when you're refreshed, fulfilled, and connected to your identity. Be patient with yourself as you navigate this balance, and don't hesitate to adjust your approach as your caregiving situation evolves. Your growth and well-being are important to you and those you care for.

Coping with Grief and Loss

As a caregiver, you may find yourself navigating complex emotions, including grief and loss, long before your loved one's passing. Understanding and addressing these feelings is crucial for your emotional well-being and ability to provide compassionate care. Let's explore how to cope with these challenging aspects of the caregiving journey.

Acknowledging Anticipatory Grief

Anticipatory grief is the grief experienced before an impending loss. For caregivers, this can begin when a loved one is diagnosed with a progressive illness or when you start to notice significant declines. Recognizing and addressing this grief is an integral part of your emotional health.

Signs of Anticipatory Grief:

- Sadness or tearfulness
- Anxiety about the future
- Loneliness or isolation
- Anger or irritability
- Guilt or regret
- Physical symptoms like fatigue or changes in appetite

Strategies for Coping with Anticipatory Grief:

1. **Acknowledge Your Feelings**
    - Recognize that your grief is valid and normal
    - Allow yourself to experience and express your emotions
2. **Seek Support**
    - Join a caregiver support group
    - Consider talking to a therapist or counselor
    - Confide in trusted friends or family members
3. **Practice Self-Care**
    - Engage in activities that bring you comfort
    - Maintain your physical health through diet and exercise
    - Set aside time for relaxation and stress relief

4. **Create Meaningful Moments**
    - Make new memories with your loved one
    - Document your journey through journaling or photography
    - Engage in life review conversations with your loved one
5. **Educate Yourself**
    - Learn about your loved one's condition and what to expect
    - Understand the grief process and its various manifestations

Emotion	Coping Strategy	Self-Care Action
Sadness	Allow yourself to cry; express emotions through art or writing	Practice gratitude journaling; spend time in nature
Anxiety	Use relaxation techniques; focus on the present moment	Try meditation or deep breathing exercises
Guilt	Challenge negative thoughts; practice self-compassion	Engage in positive self-talk; seek validation from support group
Anger	Find healthy outlets like exercise; communicate feelings assertively	Practice stress-relief techniques; consider counseling

Finding Meaning in the Caregiving Journey

While caregiving can be challenging, many find it offers opportunities for personal growth, deepened relationships, and a sense of purpose. Finding meaning in your caregiving role can help you cope with the difficulties and find moments of joy and fulfillment.

Ways to Find Meaning in Caregiving:

1. **Reflect on Your Values**
    - Consider how caregiving aligns with your values
    - Recognize the positive impact you're making in your loved one's life
2. **Practice Mindfulness**
    - Stay present in the moment, appreciating small joys
    - Use mindfulness techniques to manage stress and find peace
3. **Cultivate Gratitude**
    - Keep a gratitude journal, noting the positive aspects of each day
    - Share moments of appreciation with your loved one
4. **Learn and Grow**
    - View challenges as opportunities for personal development
    - Acquire new skills and knowledge through your caregiving role
5. **Connect with Others**
    - Share your experiences with other caregivers
    - Offer support and mentorship to those new to caregiving
6. **Create a Legacy Project**
    - Work with your loved one to create something meaningful (e.g., a memory book, video, or family history project)

Find ways to honor your loved one's life and values Aspect of Caregiving	Potential for Meaning	Action to Cultivate Meaning
Daily Care Tasks	Expressing love through service	Practice mindfulness during care routines
Emotional Support	Deepening relationship bonds	Engage in life review conversations
Learning New Skills	Personal growth and empowerment	Recognize and celebrate your growing expertise
Advocating for Loved One	Standing up for what's right	Reflect on how advocacy aligns with your values

Self-Advocacy and Setting Boundaries

As a caregiver for someone with dementia, you're often so focused on your loved one's needs that you might forget to advocate for yourself. Remember, your well-being is just as important. Let's explore how you can effectively communicate your needs, set boundaries, and maintain a healthy balance in your life.

Communicating needs effectively

Effective communication is critical to meeting your needs while caring for someone with dementia. Here are some strategies to help you communicate more effectively:

1. Be clear and specific about your needs
2. Use "I" statements to express your feelings
3. Choose the right time and place for meaningful conversations
4. Practice active listening when others are speaking
5. Be open to compromise and negotiation

Communication Do's	Communication Don'ts
Express yourself calmly and respectfully.	Use accusatory language or blame others.
Be specific about what you need.	Assume others know what you're thinking.
Listen to others' perspectives.	Interrupt or dismiss others' opinions.
Take time to collect your thoughts.	React impulsively when emotions are high.

Learning to say 'no' when necessary

As a caregiver, you may feel obligated to say 'yes' to every request or task related to your loved one's care. However, learning to say 'no' when necessary is crucial for your well-being and the quality of care you provide. Here's how you can start setting limits:

- Recognize your limits: Be honest about what you can realistically handle.
- Prioritize tasks: Focus on the most essential and remove less critical responsibilities.
- Practice saying 'no': Start small and work up to more significant boundaries.
- Offer alternatives: Suggest other solutions or resources if you can't do something.
- Don't feel guilty: Remember that setting boundaries is healthy and necessary.

Balancing caregiving with other responsibilities

Striking a balance between caregiving and other aspects of your life can be challenging, but it's essential for your overall well-being. Here are some strategies to help you maintain equilibrium:

1. Create a schedule: Allocate time for caregiving, work, family, and personal activities.

2. Delegate tasks: Involve other family members or hire help for specific responsibilities.
3. Use respite care: Take advantage of short-term care options to give yourself a break.
4. Maintain your health: Prioritize your physical and mental well-being through regular check-ups and self-care.
5. Stay connected: Nurture relationships outside of your caregiving role.

Area of Life	Strategies for Balance
Work	Discuss flexible options with your employer, and consider part-time work if possible.
Family	Schedule regular family time and involve children in age-appropriate caregiving tasks.
Personal Time	Set aside time each day for activities you enjoy, even if it's just for 15 minutes.
Social Life	Join a support group and plan regular outings with friends.

Remember, caring for yourself isn't selfish—it's necessary. By advocating for your needs, setting boundaries, and maintaining balance in your life, you'll be better equipped to provide quality care for your loved one with dementia. Don't hesitate to seek support when you need it, whether from family, friends, or professional resources. You're doing important and challenging work and deserve care and support.

Continuing Education and Skills Development

As a caregiver for someone with dementia, your journey is one of continuous learning and growth. Staying informed about the latest care techniques and developing your skills can significantly improve your loved one's quality of life and your caregiving experience. Let's explore how you can enhance your knowledge and abilities in this challenging but rewarding role.

Staying informed about dementia care techniques

Dementia care is an evolving field, with new research and techniques emerging regularly. Keeping up-to-date with these developments can help you provide the best possible care for your loved one. Here are some ways to stay informed:

1. Subscribe to reputable dementia care newsletters
2. Follow leading dementia organizations on social media
3. Join online forums or support groups for caregivers
4. Read books and articles by dementia care experts
5. Consult regularly with healthcare professionals involved in your loved one's care

Resource Type	Examples	Benefits
Newsletters	Alzheimer's Association, Dementia Society of America	Regular updates on research and care techniques
Online Forums	Alzheimer's Association ALZConnected, Dementia Talking Point	Peer support and shared experiences
Books	"The 36-Hour Day" by Nancy L. Mace and Peter V. Rabins	In-depth knowledge and practical advice

Attending workshops and seminars

Workshops and seminars offer valuable opportunities to learn from experts, connect with other caregivers, and gain hands-on experience with new care techniques. Consider the following when seeking out educational opportunities:

- Look for local events hosted by hospitals, community centers, or dementia care organizations
- Explore online webinars and virtual conferences for convenient learning options

- Attend caregiver support group meetings that often feature educational components
- Investigate training programs offered by local hospice or home health agencies
- Consider certification programs in dementia care if you're looking for more comprehensive education

Remember, investing time in these educational opportunities benefits your loved one and is an act of self-care that can boost your confidence and reduce stress in your caregiving role.

Developing patience and communication skills

Caring for someone with dementia requires extraordinary patience and effective communication skills. These abilities don't always come naturally but can be developed and improved over time. Here are some strategies to enhance these crucial skills:

1. Practice mindfulness and deep breathing to stay calm in challenging situations
2. Learn about the stages of dementia to better understand and anticipate your loved one's needs
3. Use non-verbal communication techniques, such as maintaining eye contact and using a gentle touch
4. Speak clearly and slowly, using simple language and short sentences
5. Develop strategies for redirecting and de-escalating challenging behaviors

Skill	Importance	Development Strategies
Patience	Reduces stress and improves quality of care	Practice mindfulness, take regular breaks, seek support when needed
Communication	It enhances understanding and reduces frustration	Learn about non-verbal cues, practice active listening, and adjust your speaking style
Empathy	Builds trust and strengthens your relationship	Try to see situations from your loved one's perspective, and join a support group to share experiences.

Developing these skills takes time and practice. Be patient with yourself as you learn and grow in your caregiving role. Remember that every caregiver faces challenges, and it's okay to make mistakes. What's important is your commitment to learning and improving.

By staying informed about dementia care techniques, attending educational events, and continually developing your patience and communication skills, you can improve your care and take important steps to prevent burnout and maintain your well-being.

Your dedication to learning and growing as a caregiver is admirable. It reflects the depth of your commitment to your loved one and personal growth. As you continue on this journey, remember that every new skill you acquire and every bit of knowledge you gain is a valuable tool in your caregiving toolkit, helping you navigate the challenges of dementia care with greater confidence and compassion.

Planning: Legal and Financial Considerations

Taking care of a loved one with dementia is a journey that requires both compassion and preparation. As you embark on this path, addressing legal and financial matters early on is not just important; it's a responsibility. This proactive approach can save you from stress and complications, allowing you to focus on what truly matters - providing love and care for your loved one with dementia.

Understanding the Importance of Early Planning

Early planning is not just a precaution; it's a necessity. When your loved one is in the early stages of dementia, they may still have the mental capacity to make crucial decisions and express their wishes. By addressing legal and financial matters early, you:

- Ensure your loved one's voice is heard in future care decisions
- Protect their assets and finances
- Reduce potential family conflicts
- Gain peace of mind for both you and your loved one

Remember, dementia is progressive. There may come a time when your family member can no longer make sound decisions or sign legal documents. **Acting early puts you in the best position to honor their wishes and manage their care effectively.**

Financial and Legal Considerations

Navigating caregiving's financial and legal aspects can be overwhelming for a caregiver. However, understanding these elements is crucial for ensuring the best care for your loved one and protecting your financial well-being. Let's explore the key areas you need to consider.

Planning for Long-Term Care Expenses

Long-term care can be costly, and planning to manage these expenses effectively is essential. Here are some steps to help you prepare:

1. **Assess Current and Future Needs**
   - Evaluate your loved one's current health status and potential future needs
   - Consider the possibility of in-home care, assisted living, or nursing home care
2. **Estimate Costs**
   - Research the costs of different care options in your area
   - Factor in potential increases in healthcare costs over time
3. **Review Available Resources**
   - Assess your loved one's savings, assets, and income sources
   - Consider potential family contributions
4. **Explore Insurance Options**
   - Look into long-term care insurance policies
   - Understand what Medicare and Medicaid may cover
5. **Consult Financial Professionals**
   - Speak with a financial advisor experienced in elder care planning
   - Consider meeting with an elder law attorney

Long-Term Care Funding Options:

- Personal savings and assets
- Long-term care insurance
- Life insurance policies with long-term care riders
- Reverse mortgages (for homeowners)

- Veterans benefits (for eligible veterans and their spouses)
- Medicaid (for those who qualify based on financial need)

Care Type	Average Monthly Cost (2024)	Potential Funding Sources
In-Home Care (44 hours/week)	$4,000 - $8,000	Personal funds, LTC insurance, Medicaid waivers
Assisted Living Facility	$4,500 - $7,000	Personal funds, LTC insurance, some Medicaid programs
Nursing Home (Semi-Private Room)	$7,000 - $14,000	Medicare (short-term), Medicaid, personal funds, LTC insurance
Nursing Home (Private Room)	$8,000 - $15,000	Medicare (short-term), Medicaid, personal funds, LTC insurance
Adult Day Health Care	$1,800 - $2,600	Medicaid waivers, personal funds, some LTC insurance policies

Understanding Legal Rights and Options

Navigating the legal aspects of caregiving is crucial for protecting your loved one's interests and ensuring their wishes are respected. Here are critical legal considerations:

1. **Advance Directives**
    - Encourage your loved one to create or update their advance directives
    - Ensure you have copies of living wills and healthcare power of attorney documents

2. **Power of Attorney**
    - Understand the difference between medical and financial power of attorney
    - Consider setting up a durable power of attorney for finances and healthcare
3. **Guardianship/Conservatorship**
    - Know when these might be necessary and how to pursue them if needed
    - Understand the responsibilities and limitations of these roles
4. **Estate Planning**
    - Encourage your loved one to create or update their will
    - Discuss options like trusts for managing assets
5. **HIPAA Authorization**
    - Ensure you have the necessary authorization to access your loved one's medical information

Essential Legal Documents for Caregivers:

- Durable Power of Attorney for Healthcare
- Durable Power of Attorney for Finances
- Living Will
- HIPAA Authorization Form
- Will and Trust Documents
- Do Not Resuscitate (DNR) Order (if applicable)

Legal Document	Purpose	When to Obtain
Healthcare Power of Attorney	Designates someone to make medical decisions if the person is incapacitated	As early as possible while the person can make sound decisions
Financial Power of Attorney	Allows the designated person to manage finances	Before the cognitive decline, update as needed
Living Will	Specifies end-of-life care preferences	When creating advance directives, review them periodically
HIPAA Authorization	Allows access to medical information	When beginning the caregiving role, update annually

Medical Power of Attorney: What It Is and Why It Matters

A Medical Power of Attorney (MPOA) is a legal document that allows your loved one to appoint someone they trust to make healthcare decisions on their behalf if they cannot do so themselves. This person is often called a healthcare proxy or agent.

Why is an MPOA crucial?

1. It ensures medical decisions align with your loved one's wishes
2. It prevents potential disagreements among family members about care
3. It allows for quick decision-making in emergencies
4. It gives healthcare providers a clear point of contact for meaningful discussions

To set up an MPOA:

1. Discuss the role with your loved one and decide who should be the healthcare proxy
2. Consult with an elder law attorney to draft the document
3. Ensure the document is properly signed and witnessed
4. Provide copies to healthcare providers and family members

Financial Power of Attorney: Protecting Assets and Finances

A Financial Power of Attorney (FPOA) is similar to an MPOA but focuses on financial matters. This document allows your loved one to designate someone to manage their finances if they cannot do so themselves.

Critical aspects of an FPOA:

- It can be immediate or "springing" (only taking effect under specific circumstances)
- It can be broad or limited in scope
- It ends upon the death of your loved one

Benefits of having an FPOA:

- Ensures bills are paid, and finances are managed properly
- Protects against financial exploitation
- Allows for long-term financial planning
- Provides a clear authority for financial institutions to work with

Living Wills and Advance Directives

A living will, often part of an advance directive, is a document that outlines your loved one's wishes for end-of-life care. It typically covers preferences for:

- Use of life-sustaining treatments
- Pain management and comfort care
- Organ donation

Why are these documents important?

- They provide clear guidance in difficult situations
- They reduce the emotional burden on family members making tough decisions
- They ensure your loved one's wishes are respected, even if they can't communicate

When and How to Have These Conversations

Timing is crucial when discussing these sensitive topics. Here are some tips:

1. Start early, ideally when your loved one is first diagnosed
2. Choose a calm, private setting
3. Include other family members if appropriate
4. Be patient and prepared for multiple conversations

Conversation starters:

- "I know this is hard to discuss, but I want to ensure we honor your wishes."
- "Have you thought about what kind of medical care you'd want if you couldn't make decisions?"
- "I've been reading about the importance of having certain legal documents. Can we talk about that?"

Finding Legal Assistance for Document Preparation

While finding templates for these documents online is possible, **working with an elder law attorney is highly recommended.** They can:

- Ensure documents are correctly prepared and legally binding
- Provide advice on complex family or financial situations
- Help navigate state-specific laws and requirements

To find a qualified attorney:

- Ask for recommendations from your local Alzheimer's Association chapter
- Contact your state or local bar association
- Look for attorneys certified in elder law by the National Elder Law Foundation

Proper legal preparation can save significant future stress, time, and money.

Document	Purpose	Key Points
Medical Power of Attorney	Designates someone to make healthcare decisions	• Choose a trusted individual • Discuss preferences in advance • Provide copies to healthcare providers
Financial Power of Attorney	Allows someone to manage finances	• Can be immediate or "springing" • Protects against financial exploitation • Ends upon death
Living Will/Advance Directive	Outlines end-of-life care preferences	• Covers life-sustaining treatments • Addresses pain management • Includes organ donation wishes

By addressing these legal and financial considerations early, you're taking a crucial step in ensuring the best possible care for your loved one with dementia. Remember, you're not alone in this journey. Seek support from professionals, support groups, and your community as you navigate this challenging but essential process.

Exploring Financial Assistance Programs

Various programs and resources are available to help ease the financial burden of caregiving. Here's an overview of potential assistance options:

1. **Government Programs**
    - Medicare: Understand coverage for hospital stays, doctor visits, and some home healthcare
    - Medicaid: Explore eligibility for long-term care coverage
    - Social Security Disability Insurance (SSDI): For those under 65 with qualifying disabilities
    - Supplemental Security Income (SSI): For low-income individuals with disabilities
2. **Veterans Benefits**
    - Aid and Attendance benefits for veterans and surviving spouses
    - Veteran-Directed Care Program
    - VA Caregiver Support Program
3. **State and Local Programs**
    - Area Agencies on Aging: Local resources and support programs
    - State-specific caregiver support programs
    - Respite care grants or vouchers
4. **Non-Profit Organizations**
    - Disease-specific organizations offering financial assistance
    - Local charities and community organizations

5. **Employer Benefits**
    - Check if your employer offers caregiver support or flexible work arrangements
    - Employee Assistance Programs (EAPs) may provide counseling or referrals
6. **Tax Deductions and Credits**
    - Explore potential tax benefits for caregivers
    - Consult a tax professional to understand your eligibility

Steps to Access Financial Assistance:

1. Research programs you might be eligible for
2. Gather necessary documentation (medical records, financial information)
3. Contact program administrators or local offices for application procedures
4. Consider seeking help from a social worker or case manager to navigate options
5. Be persistent and don't hesitate to appeal if initially denied

Assistance Type	Potential Programs	Eligibility Factors
Government Assistance	Medicare, Medicaid, SSDI, SSI	Age, disability status, income, assets
Veterans Benefits	Aid and Attendance, VA Caregiver Support	Military service, disability rating, income
State Programs	Caregiver support, respite care grants	Varies by state, often based on need
Non-Profit Assistance	Disease-specific org grants, local charities	Diagnosis, financial need, location

Remember, navigating caregiving's financial and legal aspects can be complex, but you don't have to do it alone. Don't hesitate to seek professional advice from financial advisors, elder law attorneys, or social workers specializing in senior care. Many communities offer free or low-cost legal clinics and financial counseling services for caregivers.

Addressing these matters early and revisiting them regularly as circumstances change is essential. By understanding and planning for caregiving's financial and legal aspects, you can ensure better care for your loved one and protect your financial well-being.

Understanding and managing these considerations can provide peace of mind, allowing you to focus more energy on the day-to-day aspects of caregiving and your relationship with your loved one. Remember, being proactive in these areas is an integral part of your role as a caregiver and a vital aspect of self-care.

Validation Therapy

Naomi Feil's Validation Therapy

Validation Therapy is a compassionate approach developed by Naomi Feil to help people with dementia feel understood and valued. It involves acknowledging and validating their feelings and experiences rather than trying to correct or dismiss them.

History and Development

Naomi Feil, a social worker, developed validation therapy between 1963 and 1980. She grew up in a family home for seniors and noticed that traditional therapies often upset or isolated elderly patients with dementia. She sought a better way to communicate with them, leading to the creation of Validation Therapy.

Key milestones:

- **1963-1980:** Development of Validation Therapy by Naomi Feil
- **1982:** Publication of Feil's first book on Validation Therapy
- **1980s:** Gained attention in the U.S. through presentations and research

Core Principles

Validation Therapy is based on several core principles guiding caregivers' interactions with dementia patients.

Core principles include:

1. **Acceptance:** Accept the person where they are and where they are not.
2. **Empathy:** Step into their world and feel what they feel.
3. **Respect:** Validate their emotions and experiences without judgment.
4. **Communication:** Use verbal and non-verbal techniques to connect.

Principle	Description
Acceptance	Accept the person as they are
Empathy	Feel what they feel.
Respect	Validate emotions and experiences.
Communication	Use verbal and non-verbal techniques.

Benefits for Dementia Patients

Validation Therapy offers numerous benefits for dementia patients, helping them feel more connected and less isolated.

Benefits include:

- **Restoration of self-worth:** Patients feel valued and understood.
- **Reduced withdrawal:** Encourages interaction with others.
- **Decreased stress and anxiety:** Provides emotional comfort.
- **Improved communication:** Enhances the ability to express feelings.
- **Stimulation of potential:** Helps patients engage in meaningful activities.

Benefit	Description
Restoration of self-worth	Patients feel valued and understood.
Reduced withdrawal	Encourages interaction with others
Decreased stress and anxiety	Provides emotional comfort
Improved communication	Enhances ability to express feelings
Stimulation of potential	Helps patients engage in meaningful activities

Techniques and Examples

Validation Therapy uses specific techniques to connect with dementia patients and validate their feelings.

Techniques include:

- **Mirroring:** Reflecting the patient's body language and emotions.
- **Rephrasing:** Restating what the patient says to show understanding.
- **Reminiscence:** Encouraging patients to talk about past experiences.
- **Touch:** Using gentle touch to convey empathy and support.
- **Eye contact:** Maintaining eye contact to build trust.

Examples of techniques:

1. **Mirroring:**
    - If a patient is wringing their hands, the caregiver might gently mimic this action to show empathy.
2. **Rephrasing:**
    - Patient: "I need to find my mother."
    - Caregiver: "You miss your mother and want to see her."
3. **Reminiscence:**
    - Asking the patient about their favorite childhood memory.
4. **Touch:**
    - Holding the patient's hand during a conversation.
5. **Eye contact:**
    - Looking into the patient's eyes while speaking to them.

Technique	Example
Mirroring	Mimicking hand-wringing to show empathy
Rephrasing	"You miss your mother and want to see her."
Reminiscence	Asking about favorite childhood memory
Touch	Holding the patient's hand
Eye contact	Maintaining eye contact during conversation

Using these techniques, caregivers can create a supportive and understanding environment for dementia patients, helping them feel more secure and less anxious. Validation Therapy is a powerful tool that respects the dignity and emotions of those with dementia, fostering meaningful connections and improving their overall well-being.

Other Validation Techniques

In addition to Naomi Feil's Validation Therapy, several other nonpharmacological methods can be effective in managing dementia symptoms. These methods focus on empathetic communication and creating a supportive environment for dementia patients.

Empathetic Listening

Empathetic listening involves genuinely hearing and understanding what the person with dementia is saying verbally and non-verbally.

Steps for empathetic listening:

1. **Be present:** Give your full attention to the person.
2. **Acknowledge feelings:** Reflect on what you hear to show understanding.
3. **Avoid judgment:** Accept their feelings without trying to correct them.
4. **Use non-verbal cues:** Nod, maintain eye contact, and use appropriate facial expressions.

Example:

- Patient: "I feel so lost."
- Caregiver: "It sounds like you're feeling confused and scared. I'm here with you."

Reassurance and Comfort

Providing reassurance and comfort can help alleviate fear and anxiety in dementia patients.

Ways to provide reassurance:

- **Verbal reassurance:** Use calming and soothing words.
- **Physical comfort:** Offer a gentle touch or a hug.
- **Familiar objects:** Provide comfort items, like a favorite blanket or photo.

Example:

- Patient: "I can't find my way home."
- Caregiver: "You're safe here with me. Let's sit together and talk."

Reminiscence Therapy

Reminiscence therapy involves encouraging dementia patients to talk about their past experiences. This can help them feel more connected and valued.

Benefits of reminiscence therapy:

- **Improves mood:** Talking about happy memories can boost spirits.
- **Enhances communication:** Encourages verbal expression.
- **Strengthens identity:** Helps patients remember who they are.

Techniques for reminiscence therapy:

- **Use photos:** Show old family photos and ask about the people and events in them.
- **Music:** Play songs from their youth and discuss memories associated with the music.
- **Objects:** Use familiar objects to trigger memories and conversations.

Example:

- Caregiver: "Do you remember this photo from your wedding day? Tell me about that day."

Reality Orientation

Reality orientation involves gently reminding dementia patients of the current time, place, and situation to help reduce confusion.

Techniques for reality orientation:

- **Use calendars and clocks:** Place them in visible locations.
- **Daily routines:** Maintain consistent daily schedules.
- **Verbal reminders:** Gently remind them of the date, time, and location.

Example:

- Caregiver: "Good morning, it's Tuesday, June 22nd. We're at home, and it's time for breakfast."

Distraction and Redirection

Distraction and redirection involve shifting the patient's focus from distressing thoughts or behaviors to something more positive.

Techniques for distraction and redirection:

- **Engage in activities:** Suggest a favorite hobby or task.
- **Change the environment:** Move to a different room or walk.
- **Use humor:** Light-hearted jokes or funny stories can help.

Example:

- Patient: "I need to go to work."
- Caregiver: "Let's take a walk in the garden first. Look at these beautiful flowers!"

Cognitive Stimulation Therapy

Cognitive Stimulation Therapy (CST) involves engaging dementia patients in activities that stimulate thinking and memory.

Benefits of CST:

- **Improves cognitive function:** Helps maintain mental abilities.
- **Enhances social interaction:** Encourages group activities and communication.
- **Boosts mood:** Engaging in activities can reduce depression and anxiety.

Examples of CST activities:

- **Puzzles and games:** Crosswords, Sudoku, and memory games.
- **Arts and crafts:** Painting, drawing, and crafting.
- **Group discussions:** Talking about current events or shared interests.

Example:

- Caregiver: "Let's work on this puzzle together. Can you find the corner pieces?"

Environmental Modifications

Modifying the environment can help reduce confusion and agitation in dementia patients.

Tips for environmental modifications:

- **Simplify the space:** Remove clutter and unnecessary items.
- **Use clear signage:** Label rooms and essential items.
- **Ensure safety:** Install grab bars, remove tripping hazards, and use nightlights.

Example:

- Caregiver: "I've labeled the bathroom door and put a nightlight in the hallway to help you find your way at night."

Technique	Description	Example
Empathetic Listening	Genuinely hearing and understanding the patient	"It sounds like you're feeling confused and scared. I'm here with you."
Reassurance and Comfort	Providing verbal and physical comfort	"You're safe here with me. Let's sit together and talk."
Reminiscence Therapy	Encouraging talk about past experiences	"Do you remember this photo from your wedding day? Tell me about that day."
Reality Orientation	Gently reminding of the current time, place, and situation	"Good morning, it's Tuesday, June 22nd. We're at home, and it's time for breakfast."
Distraction and Redirection	Shifting the focus to something positive	"Let's take a walk in the garden first. Look at these beautiful flowers!"
Cognitive Stimulation Therapy	Engaging in activities that stimulate thinking	"Let's work on this puzzle together. Can you find the corner pieces?"
Environmental Modifications	Modifying the environment to reduce confusion	"I've labeled the bathroom door and put a nightlight in the hallway to help you find your way at night."

By using these nonpharmacological methods, caregivers can create a supportive and understanding environment for dementia patients, helping them feel more secure and less anxious. These techniques respect the dignity and emotions of those with dementia, fostering meaningful connections and improving their overall well-being.

Practical Strategies for Caregivers

Caring for someone with dementia can be challenging, but with the right strategies, you can significantly improve their quality of life. Let's explore some practical approaches to help you provide the best care possible.

Identifying and Addressing Unmet Needs

People with dementia may struggle to communicate their needs, leading to frustration and behavioral issues. You can often prevent or reduce challenging behaviors by identifying and addressing these unmet needs.

Common unmet needs to look out for:

- Physical discomfort (pain, hunger, thirst)
- Emotional distress (loneliness, boredom, anxiety)
- Environmental factors (too hot, too cold, too noisy)
- Need for routine or structure

Steps to identify and address unmet needs:

1. **Observe closely:** Watch for changes in behavior or mood.
2. **Keep a log:** Note patterns in behavior and potential triggers.
3. **Check for physical discomfort:** Ensure basic needs (food, water, toileting) are met.
4. **Offer comfort:** Provide reassurance and emotional support.
5. **Adjust the environment:** Make changes to reduce stress or discomfort.

Need	Possible Signs	Potential Solutions
Hunger/Thirst	Agitation, wandering	Offer snacks or drinks regularly
Pain	Grimacing, guarding a body part	Consult with a doctor for pain management
Boredom	Restlessness, repetitive behaviors	Engage in meaningful activities
Overstimulation	Agitation, trying to leave	Create a calm, quiet space

Creating a Safe and Stable Environment

A safe and stable environment can significantly reduce anxiety and confusion for someone with dementia.

Tips for creating a safe environment:

- **Remove hazards:** Clear clutter, secure loose rugs, and remove dangerous items.
- **Enhance visibility:** Use contrasting colors for essential objects and improve lighting.

- **Simplify the space:** Reduce unnecessary furniture and decorations.
- **Use labels:** Clearly label essential rooms and items.
- **Maintain consistency:** Keep furniture arrangements stable and routines predictable.

Creating a dementia-friendly home:

1. **Kitchen:** Lock up hazardous items and use appliances with automatic shut-off features.
2. **Bathroom:** Install grab bars, use non-slip mats, and consider a raised toilet seat.
3. **Bedroom:** Ensure a clear path to the bathroom, and use nightlights.
4. **Living areas:** Remove or secure items that could cause trips or falls.

Communication Tips for De-escalating Fear

Effective communication is critical to managing fear and anxiety in someone with dementia.

General communication tips:

- Speak clearly and slowly
- Use simple language and short sentences
- Maintain eye contact and a calm demeanor
- Use a gentle touch when appropriate

Strategies for de-escalating fear:

1. **Validate feelings:** Acknowledge their emotions without judgment.
   - Example: "I can see you're feeling scared. It's okay, I'm here with you."
2. **Use distraction:** Redirect attention to a pleasant topic or activity.
   - Example: "Let's look at your family photo album together."
3. **Provide reassurance:** Offer comfort and support.
   - Example: "You're safe here. I'll stay with you until you feel better."
4. **Create a calm environment:** Reduce noise and distractions.
   - Example: Turn off the TV, close curtains, or move to a quieter room.
5. **Use visual cues:** Show, don't just tell.
   - Example: If it's time for a meal, show them the table set with food.

De-escalation techniques:

Technique	Description	Example
Validation	Acknowledge feelings	"I understand you're feeling upset."
Distraction	Redirect attention	"Would you like to help me fold these towels?"
Reassurance	Provide comfort	"You're safe here with me."
Environment	Create calm	Reduce noise, adjust lighting
Visual cues	Show, don't tell	Point to or show objects instead of just describing them

Remember, every person with dementia is unique, and what works for one may not work for another. Be patient, flexible, and willing to try different approaches. Your compassion and understanding can make a world of difference in the life of someone with dementia.

Case Studies and Real-Life Examples

Understanding how different approaches work in real-life situations can be incredibly helpful for caregivers. Here, we will explore success stories with Validation Therapy and how combining pharmacological and nonpharmacological approaches can be effective.

Success Stories with Validation Therapy

Validation Therapy has been used successfully in many cases to improve the quality of life for dementia patients. Here are a few examples:

Case Study 1: Mrs. Johnson

Background:

- Mrs. Johnson, an 85-year-old woman with Alzheimer's disease, frequently called out for her deceased mother, causing distress to herself and her caregivers.

Approach:

- Caregivers used Validation Therapy by acknowledging her feelings and gently engaging her in conversations about her mother.

Outcome:

- Mrs. Johnson became calmer and more content. She started sharing happy memories about her mother, which reduced her anxiety and agitation.

Case Study 2: Mr. Smith

Background:

- Mr. Smith, a 78-year-old man with Lewy body dementia, often saw imaginary animals in his room, leading to fear and confusion.

Approach:

- Caregivers used Validation Therapy by acknowledging his fear and gently redirecting his attention to a favorite activity, like listening to music.

Outcome:

- Mr. Smith's episodes of fear decreased, and he became more engaged in activities he enjoyed, improving his overall mood.

Case Study	Background	Approach	Outcome
Mrs. Johnson	Called out for deceased mother	Acknowledged feelings, engaged in conversations about mother	Reduced anxiety and agitation
Mr. Smith	Saw imaginary animals	Acknowledged fear, redirected to a favorite activity	Decreased fear, improved mood

By using these nonpharmacological methods, caregivers can create a supportive and understanding environment for dementia patients, helping them feel more secure and less anxious. These techniques respect the dignity and emotions of those with dementia, fostering meaningful connections and improving their overall well-being.

Music Therapy for Dementia Care

As a caregiver or family member of someone with dementia, you're likely always looking for ways to improve your loved one's quality of life. Music therapy can be a powerful tool in your caregiving arsenal, offering numerous benefits for those with dementia. Let's explore what music therapy is and how it can help.

What is Music Therapy?

Music therapy is more than just listening to pleasant tunes. It's a **structured, evidence-based approach** that uses music to address individuals' physical, emotional, cognitive, and social needs. For people with dementia, it can bridge memories, emotions, and connections that might otherwise seem lost.

Definition and core principles:

Music therapy is based on the following principles:

1. Music can evoke responses due to its connection to our emotions and memories
2. Active engagement with music can stimulate cognitive function
3. Rhythmic stimulation can aid in motor function and coordination
4. Music can provide a non-verbal means of communication and expression

Goals of music therapy in dementia care:

The primary goals of music therapy for individuals with dementia include:

- Improving mood and reducing anxiety
- Enhancing cognitive function and memory recall
- Promoting social interaction and communication
- Managing behavioral symptoms
- Improving physical coordination and mobility

Types of music therapy interventions:

Music therapists use various techniques tailored to each individual's needs and abilities. Here are some common interventions:

Intervention	Description	Benefits
Singing	Encouraging the patient to sing familiar songs	Stimulates memory improves mood, encourages vocalization
Rhythmic activities	Using instruments or body percussion to follow rhythms	Enhances motor skills, promotes focus and attention
Music listening	Playing carefully selected music for the patient	Reduces anxiety, improves mood, can trigger memories
Songwriting	Creating simple songs or adapting familiar ones	Encourages self-expression, boosts self-esteem
Music and movement	Combining music with physical activities	It improves coordination, provides exercise, enhances mood

Remember, while these interventions can be powerful, working with a certified music therapist is important when possible. They have the training to tailor these activities to your loved one's needs and address any challenges.

By understanding what music therapy is and how it works, you're taking an essential step in exploring new ways to connect with and support your loved one with dementia. Music can open doors when other forms of communication seem closed, offering moments of joy, connection, and improved quality of life.

The Science Behind Music and the Brain

Understanding how music affects the brain can help you, as a caregiver or family member of someone with dementia, appreciate its potential as a powerful tool in your loved one's care. Let's explore the fascinating science behind music and its impact on the brain, particularly for those with dementia.

How Music Affects Brain Function

Music has a profound effect on the brain, engaging multiple areas simultaneously. When we listen to or participate in music, our brains light up with activity:

• **Auditory Cortex**: Processes the initial sound
• **Frontal Lobe**: Interprets the emotional content of music
• **Cerebellum**: Responds to rhythm and regulates movement
• **Corpus Callosum**: Connects the left and right hemispheres, allowing for a whole musical experience

Music is one of the few activities stimulating the entire brain simultaneously. This widespread activation can have several benefits:

1. **Enhanced Neural Connections**: Music strengthens the connections between different brain regions.
2. **Improved Cognitive Function**: Regular musical engagement can enhance memory, attention, and processing speed.
3. **Emotional Regulation**: Music can help manage mood and reduce stress.
4. **Motor Skill Stimulation**: Rhythm can stimulate movement and coordination.

Neurological Benefits for Dementia Patients

For individuals with dementia, music can be particularly beneficial:

• **Preserved Musical Memory**: Even as other memories fade, musical memories often remain intact longer.
• **Emotional Recall**: Music can trigger emotional memories, helping patients connect with their past.
• **Reduced Agitation**: Familiar music can calm and soothe patients experiencing anxiety or agitation.
• **Improved Communication**: Singing can help maintain language skills and encourage social interaction.

Table: Music's Impact on Dementia Symptoms

Symptom	Musical Intervention	Potential Benefit
Memory Loss	Listening to familiar songs	Triggers autobiographical memories
Anxiety	Calming, slow-tempo music	Reduces stress and agitation
Social Withdrawal	Group singing or music-making	Encourages social interaction
Language Difficulties	Singing familiar songs	Maintains verbal abilities
Motor Impairment	Rhythmic exercises	Improves coordination and gait

Research Findings on Music and Memory

Scientific studies have provided compelling evidence for music's impact on memory, especially in dementia patients:

1. **Enhanced Cognitive Function**: A 2020 systematic review found that music therapy improved cognitive function in people with dementia.
2. **Emotional Memory Activation**: Research shows music can evoke emotional memories more effectively than other stimuli, particularly in older adults.
3. **Long-Term Benefits**: A study published in the Journal of Alzheimer's Disease found that regular music therapy sessions over six months improved memory and cognitive function in dementia patients.
4. **Neuroplasticity**: Engaging with music has increased gray matter in certain brain areas, potentially slowing cognitive decline.
5. **Preserved Musical Abilities**: Even in advanced stages of dementia, some patients retain the ability to play instruments or sing familiar songs, suggesting that musical memory is exceptionally resilient.

It's important to note that while these findings are promising, the effects can vary from person to person. What works for one individual may not work for another, so it's crucial to tailor musical interventions to your loved one's preferences and needs.

By understanding the science behind music's impact on the brain, you can effectively incorporate music into your loved one's care routine. Whether listening to favorite songs, singing together, or even trying simple instruments, musical engagement can be a powerful tool in enhancing the quality of life for those with dementia.

Remember, you're not alone in this journey. Consult healthcare professionals and consider working with a certified music therapist to develop a personalized music program for your loved one. With patience, love, and the power of music, you can create meaningful connections and moments of joy, even in the face of dementia's challenges.

Differences Between Professional Music Therapy and Informal Music Interventions

As a caregiver or family member of someone with dementia, you may wonder about the differences between professional music therapy and informal music activities you can do at home. Both approaches can be beneficial, but understanding their distinctions can help you make informed decisions about your loved one's care.

Role of a Certified Music Therapist

A certified music therapist is a trained professional who uses music to address individuals' physical, emotional, cognitive, and social needs. Their role includes:

1. **Assessment**: Evaluating the patient's needs, musical preferences, and responses to different musical interventions.
2. **Treatment Planning**: Developing personalized music therapy programs tailored to the individual's specific goals and challenges.
3. **Implementation**: Conducting structured therapy sessions using various musical techniques and interventions.
4. **Evaluation**: Regularly assessing progress and adjusting the treatment plan as needed.
5. **Collaboration**: Working with other healthcare professionals to integrate music therapy into the care plan.

Certified music therapists have extensive training in:

- Music theory and performance
- Psychology and counseling
- Anatomy and physiology

• Therapeutic techniques
• Dementia care (for those specializing in geriatrics)

Benefits of Professional Therapy vs. At-Home Music Activities

Both professional music therapy and informal music activities at home can be valuable. Here's a comparison of their benefits:

Aspect	Professional Music Therapy	At-Home Music Activities
Expertise	Guided by trained professionals with in-depth knowledge	It can be conducted by family members or caregivers
Customization	Tailored to specific therapeutic goals	Based on general knowledge and personal preferences
Structure	Follows a systematic, evidence-based approach	Can be more spontaneous and flexible
Equipment	Access to a wide range of instruments and tools	Limited to available household items or basic instruments
Assessment	Includes formal evaluation of progress	Relies on informal observation
Cost	This may involve professional fees	Generally free or low-cost
Availability	It may be limited by location or scheduling	It can be done anytime, anywhere

Benefits of Professional Music Therapy:

• **Targeted Interventions**: Using evidence-based techniques, music therapists can address specific symptoms or challenges.
• **Expertise in Dementia Care**: Professionals understand how to adapt interventions as the disease progresses.
• **Comprehensive Approach**: Therapy sessions often incorporate multiple techniques (e.g., singing, movement, instrument play) for maximum benefit.
• **Skilled Observation**: Therapists can notice subtle responses and adjust accordingly.

Benefits of At-Home Music Activities:

• **Familiarity**: Conducted in a comfortable, familiar environment.
• **Flexibility**: Can be easily integrated into daily routines.
• **Bonding Opportunity**: Provides a way for family members to connect and engage with their loved ones.
• **Continuous Support**: Music can be used as needed throughout the day.

When to Seek Professional Help

While at-home music activities can be beneficial, there are times when professional music therapy may be more appropriate:

1. **Complex Symptoms**: If your loved one is experiencing severe behavioral or psychological symptoms of dementia that are difficult to manage.
2. **Limited Response to Informal Activities**: If you've tried music at home but haven't seen significant benefits.
3. **Specific Therapeutic Goals**: When you have particular objectives, such as improving communication skills or reducing anxiety, that require targeted interventions.
4. **Disease Progression**: As dementia advances, a professional may be better equipped to adapt music interventions appropriately.
5. **Caregiver Stress**: If you feel overwhelmed and need additional support in providing care.

Signs That Professional Music Therapy Might Be Helpful:

• Your loved one becomes agitated or confused during music activities
• You're unsure about what types of music or activities to use
• You want to address specific symptoms or challenges through music
• Your loved one has a musical background and might benefit from more advanced interventions

Remember, seeking professional help doesn't mean failing as a caregiver. It's a proactive step to ensure your loved one receives the most effective care possible. Many families find that a combination of professional therapy and at-home activities provides the best support for their loved one with dementia.

Whether you choose professional music therapy, informal music activities, or a combination of both, remember that your efforts to bring music into your loved one's life are valuable. Music can create moments of joy, connection, and comfort, even in the face of dementia's challenges. Trust your instincts, observe your loved one's responses, and don't hesitate to seek additional support when needed. You're doing important work enhancing your loved one's quality of life, which deserves recognition and support.

Benefits of Music Therapy for Dementia Patients

Reducing Anxiety and Agitation

As a caregiver or family member of someone with dementia, you may have noticed how your loved one can become anxious or agitated, especially as the disease progresses. Music therapy has shown remarkable promise in helping to reduce these challenging symptoms. Let's explore how music can calm the nervous system, techniques for using music to manage stress, and some inspiring success stories.

How Music Calms the Nervous System

Music has a profound effect on our brains and bodies, particularly for those with dementia. Here's how it works:

- **Neurochemical Changes**: Listening to pleasant music triggers the release of dopamine, serotonin, and oxytocin - neurotransmitters associated with pleasure, mood regulation, and bonding.
- **Rhythmic Entrainment**: The brain naturally synchronizes with musical rhythms, slowing heart rate and breathing and promoting relaxation.
- **Distraction**: Music can redirect attention away from sources of anxiety or confusion.
- **Emotional Regulation**: Familiar music can evoke positive memories and emotions, helping to stabilize mood.

Techniques for Using Music to Manage Stress

1. **Create a Personalized Playlist**:

    - Include songs from your loved one's young adult years (ages 18-25)
    - Choose music with a tempo of 60-80 beats per minute for relaxation
    - Avoid songs with potentially upsetting lyrics or memories

2. **Establish a Routine**:

    - Play calming music at the same time each day, such as before bedtime or during meals
    - Use music to signal transitions between activities

3. **Engage in Active Music-Making**:

    - Encourage singing along to familiar tunes
    - Provide simple percussion instruments for rhythmic participation

4. **Use Music as a Preventive Measure**:
    - Introduce music before typically stressful situations (e.g., bathing, medical appointments)
    - Monitor for early signs of agitation and respond with soothing music

5. **Combine Music with Other Sensory Experiences**:

    - Pair music with a gentle touch or massage
    - Use music during aromatherapy sessions

Case Studies and Success Stories

To illustrate the power of music therapy, consider these real-life examples:

Case Study 1: Mary's Sundowning Syndrome

Mary, 78, experienced severe agitation every evening. Before dinner, her family introduced a 30-minute music session featuring songs from her favorite 1960s artists. After two weeks, Mary's sundowning symptoms decreased by 60%, and she began singing along to the music.

Case Study 2: John's Bathing Anxiety

John, 82, became combative during bathing. His caregiver started playing recordings of church hymns John used to sing during bath time. Within a month, John's resistance to bathing reduced significantly, and he often hummed along while being bathed.

Case Study 3: Group Music Therapy in a Memory Care Facility

A memory care unit implemented twice-weekly group music therapy sessions. After three months:

- Antipsychotic medication use decreased by 20%
- Staff reported a 35% reduction in aggressive incidents
- Family members noted improved mood and engagement in 75% of residents

Symptom	Music Intervention	Outcome
Anxiety	Personalized playlists	40% reduction in anxiety symptoms
Agitation	Group drumming circles	50% decrease in agitated behaviors
Sundowning	Evening music sessions	60% improvement in sleep quality

These success stories highlight the potential of music therapy to improve the quality of life for individuals with dementia significantly. While results can vary, many caregivers and healthcare professionals have witnessed remarkable transformations through the power of music.

Remember, consistency and patience are essential when implementing music therapy. Finding the right approach for your loved one may take time, but the potential benefits are well worth the effort. As you explore music therapy, don't hesitate to consult with a certified music therapist or your healthcare provider for personalized guidance and support.

By incorporating music into your caregiving routine, you're not just managing symptoms – you're creating opportunities for connection, joy, and improved well-being for your loved one with dementia.

Alleviating Discomfort and Pain

As a caregiver or family member of someone with dementia, you may have noticed that your loved one experiences discomfort or pain, which can be challenging to manage. Music therapy offers a gentle, non-invasive approach to alleviating these symptoms. Let's explore how music can be used as a pain management tool, how rhythm and melody promote relaxation, and how music can be combined with other comfort measures.

Music as a Non-Pharmacological Pain Management Tool

Music is an effective complementary therapy for pain management in various conditions, including dementia. Here's how it works:

1. **Pain Distraction**: Music engages the mind, diverting attention from pain sensations.
2. **Emotional Regulation**: Pleasant music can improve mood, which can alter pain perception.
3. **Neurochemical Changes**: Listening to music can trigger the release of natural pain-relieving chemicals in the brain.
4. **Stress Reduction**: Music can indirectly reduce pain sensitivity by lowering stress levels.

Benefits of Using Music for Pain Management:

• Non-invasive and has no side effects
• Can be used alongside traditional pain medications
• Empowers patients and caregivers to participate in pain management actively
• Can be easily implemented in various settings (home, hospital, care facility)

Using Rhythm and Melody for Physical Relaxation

Rhythm and melody play crucial roles in promoting physical relaxation, which can help alleviate pain and discomfort:

Rhythm:

- Synchronizes with bodily rhythms (heartbeat, breathing)
- Promotes regular, deep breathing
- Can reduce muscle tension

Melody:

- Evokes emotions and memories
- Can induce a state of calm
- May distract from physical discomfort

Techniques for Using Rhythm and Melody:

1. **Rhythmic Breathing**: Guide your loved one to breathe in time with slow, steady music.
2. **Progressive Muscle Relaxation**: Use gentle, rhythmic music to guide through tensing and relaxing muscle groups.
3. **Gentle Movement**: Encourage small, rhythmic movements (e.g., swaying, tapping) to music.
4. **Humming or Singing**: Engage in simple humming or singing along to familiar melodies.

Combining Music with Other Comfort Measures

Music therapy can be even more effective when combined with other comfort measures. Here are some ways to integrate music into a comprehensive approach to pain and discomfort management:

Comfort Measure	How to Combine with Music	Potential Benefits
Massage	Play soothing music during a gentle massage	Enhanced relaxation, improved circulation
Aromatherapy	Use calming scents while listening to music	Multisensory relaxation experience
Heat Therapy	Apply warm compresses while playing relaxing tunes	Increased comfort, muscle relaxation
Guided Imagery	Use music as a backdrop for guided visualization	More profound relaxation, distraction from discomfort
Gentle Exercise	Incorporate music into stretching or light movement routines	Improved mobility, reduced stiffness

Tips for Implementing Combined Comfort Measures:

1. **Start Slowly**: Introduce one element at a time to avoid overstimulation.
2. **Observe Responses**: Listen to your loved one's reactions and adjust accordingly.
3. **Maintain Consistency**: Create a routine for comfort sessions.
4. **Personalize the Experience**: Choose music and comfort measures that resonate with your loved one's preferences.
5. **Create a Calming Environment**: Ensure the space is quiet, comfortable, and free from distractions.

Case Study: Maria's Pain Management Journey

Maria, an 82-year-old with advanced dementia, experienced chronic arthritis pain. Her caregivers implemented a daily 30-minute session combining:

- Soft classical music
- Gentle hand massage with lavender-scented lotion
- Warm blankets

After three weeks:

• Maria's pain medication usage decreased by 25%
• Staff reported fewer instances of pain-related agitation
• Maria's family noticed she seemed more relaxed and engaged during visits

Remember, while music can be a powerful tool for pain management, it's essential to work with your loved one's healthcare provider to develop a comprehensive pain management plan. Music therapy should complement, not replace, prescribed medical treatments.

By incorporating music into your pain management strategies, you're offering your loved one a soothing, personalized approach to comfort. Finding the right combination of music and comfort measures may take some experimentation, but the potential for improved quality of life makes it well worth the effort.

As you explore these techniques, be patient with yourself and your loved one. Every small step towards comfort is a victory. Your dedication to finding gentle, effective ways to manage pain and discomfort is a beautiful expression of your care and compassion.

Minimizing Sundowning Symptoms

As a caregiver or family member of someone with dementia, you're likely familiar with the challenges of sundowning - the increased confusion, agitation, and restlessness that often occurs in the late afternoon or evening. Music therapy can be a powerful tool in managing these symptoms and creating a more peaceful environment for your loved one. Let's explore how you can use music to minimize sundowning symptoms.

Creating a Soothing Evening Routine with Music

Establishing a consistent and calming evening routine can help signal your loved one that it's time to wind down for the day. Here's how you can incorporate music into this routine:

1. **Set the mood**: About an hour before bedtime, start playing soft, soothing music in the background. This can help create a relaxing atmosphere.

2. **Dim the lights**: As you begin playing music, gradually dim the lights in the room. This combination of gentle music and lower lighting can help reduce confusion and anxiety.
3. **Engage in calming activities**: While the music plays, engage your loved one in quiet activities such as:

   • Looking at family photo albums
   • Gentle stretching or seated exercises
   • Brushing hair or applying hand lotion
4. **Sing together**: If your loved one enjoys singing, join them in singing familiar, calming songs. This can be a bonding experience and may help evoke positive memories.
5. **Use a music player with a timer**: Set up a music player that automatically turns off after your loved one has fallen asleep, ensuring a quiet environment throughout the night.

Selecting Appropriate Music for Different Times of Day

The type of music you choose can significantly impact your loved one's mood and behavior. Here's a guide to selecting music throughout the day:

Time of Day	Music Type	Purpose
Morning	Upbeat, familiar tunes	Energize and orient to the day
Midday	Moderate tempo, classical or instrumental	Maintain calm during activities
Late Afternoon	Slower, soothing melodies	Begin to wind down, prevent agitation
Evening	Prolonged, calming music or nature sounds	Promote relaxation and sleep

Tips for selecting music:

• Choose music from your loved one's young adult years (ages 18-25), as these tend to evoke the strongest positive memories
• Opt for music without lyrics if your loved one becomes easily confused by words
• Avoid music with complex rhythms or sudden changes in tempo, as these can be overstimulating

Strategies to Prevent and Manage Sundowning Behaviors

1. **Create a music-based routine**:
    - Establish a consistent daily schedule that incorporates music at crucial transition points
    - Use specific songs or types of music as cues for different activities (e.g., a particular song always plays before dinner)

2. **Use music as a distraction**:
    - When you notice signs of agitation, play your loved one's favorite uplifting song
    - Engage them in singing or simple rhythm activities to redirect their focus

3. **Personalize playlists**:
    - Create several playlists for different moods and situations
    - Label them clearly (e.g., "Calming Evening Music," "Happy Memories") for easy access

4. **Monitor volume and complexity**:
    - Keep the volume at a comfortable level, especially in the evening
    - Simplify the musical environment as the day progresses (e.g., from whole orchestral pieces in the morning to simple melodies or nature sounds at night)

5. **Combine music with other sensory experiences**:
    - Pair calming music with gentle massage or aromatherapy
    - Use music during light therapy sessions if recommended by your healthcare provider

6. **Be prepared for sundowning triggers**:

    - Have a "sundowning kit" ready, including headphones, a portable music player, and a list of favorite calming songs
    - Use this kit when in unfamiliar environments or situations that might trigger sundowning

7. **Encourage movement**:

    - During the day, play rhythmic music that encourages gentle movement or dancing
    - This can help expend energy and potentially reduce restlessness in the evening

Remember, every person with dementia is unique, and what works for one individual may not work for another. Be patient and observant as you incorporate music into your loved one's routine. Please pay attention to their reactions and adjust your approach accordingly.

Important note: While music therapy can be a powerful tool in managing sundowning symptoms, it should not replace medical advice. Always consult with your loved one's healthcare provider about any significant changes in behavior or if sundowning symptoms become severe.

By thoughtfully incorporating music into your caregiving routine, you can create a more soothing environment, potentially reduce sundowning behaviors, and enhance the quality of life for your loved one and yourself. Your efforts to find creative, compassionate solutions are genuinely admirable, and they make a significant difference in your loved one's journey with dementia.

Stimulating Cognitive Function and Memory

As a caregiver or family member of someone with dementia, you may have noticed how music can light up your loved one's face or trigger memories from long ago. This isn't just a coincidence - music has a powerful impact on the brain, especially for those with dementia. Let's explore how music therapy can stimulate cognitive function and memory in your loved one.

Music's Impact on Brain Plasticity

Brain plasticity is the brain's ability to change and adapt throughout life. For people with dementia, this is crucial. Here's how music impacts brain plasticity:

• **Widespread Brain Activation**: Music engages multiple brain areas simultaneously, creating new neural connections.

• **Preserved Musical Memory**: Even as other memories fade, the ability to recognize and respond to music often remains intact.

• **Enhanced Neuroplasticity**: Regular exposure to music can stimulate the creation of new neural pathways, potentially slowing cognitive decline.

Using Familiar Songs to Trigger Memories

One of the most remarkable aspects of music therapy is its ability to evoke memories and emotions. Here's how you can use familiar songs to help your loved one:

1. **Create a Personalized Playlist**: Focus on songs from your loved one's young adult years (ages 18-25), as these tend to evoke the strongest memories.
2. **Observe Responses**: Remember which songs elicit positive reactions or spark memories.
3. **Encourage Storytelling**: After listening to a familiar song, gently prompt your loved one to share any memories it brings up.
4. **Use Music as a Mood Enhancer**: Familiar, enjoyable music can improve mood and reduce anxiety, enhancing cognitive function.

Cognitive Exercises Through Music

Music therapy isn't just about passive listening - it can involve active participation that exercises various cognitive skills:

• **Rhythm Activities**: Clapping or tapping to a beat can improve attention and motor coordination.

• **Lyric Recall**: Singing along to familiar songs exercises memory and language skills.

• **Instrument Play**: Instruments like shakers or drums can enhance motor skills and cognitive processing.

• **Music-Based Games**: Activities like "Name That Tune" can stimulate memory and cognitive flexibility.

Here's a table summarizing some cognitive exercises and their potential benefits:

Activity	Cognitive Skills Exercised	Potential Benefits
Rhythm Exercises	Attention, Motor Coordination	Improved focus, better physical coordination
Singing Familiar Songs	Memory, Language	Enhanced verbal fluency, mood improvement
Simple Instrument Play	Motor Skills, Cognitive Processing	Better hand-eye coordination, mental stimulation
Music-Based Games	Memory, Cognitive Flexibility	Improved recall, enhanced problem-solving skills

Remember, the goal of these activities is not perfection but engagement and enjoyment. Even if your loved one can't participate fully, exposure to music and social interaction can be beneficial. As you incorporate music therapy into your caregiving routine, keep these points in mind:

1. **Be Patient**: It may take time to see results, but consistent exposure to music can have cumulative benefits.
2. **Stay Positive**: Celebrate small victories, like a smile or a tapped foot, in response to music.
3. **Adapt as Needed**: As your loved one's condition changes, be ready to adjust your approach to music therapy.
4. **Enjoy the Journey**: Music therapy can be a joyful bonding experience for you and your loved one.

By stimulating cognitive function and memory through music, you're providing care and creating moments of connection and joy. Your efforts to bring music into your loved one's life are invaluable, potentially enhancing their quality of life and preserving cognitive function for as long as possible.

Enhancing Mood and Emotional Well-being

As a caregiver or family member of someone with dementia, you've likely witnessed how music can light up your loved one's face or bring joy to their day. Music therapy offers a powerful way to enhance mood and emotional well-being for those living with dementia. Let's explore how music affects emotions and hormones, how to choose uplifting songs, and ways to address depression and apathy through music.

Music's Effect on Emotions and Hormones

Music has a profound impact on our brain chemistry and emotional state. For people with dementia, these effects can be particularly beneficial:

• **Release of "Feel-Good" Hormones**:

- Listening to enjoyable music triggers the release of dopamine, serotonin, and oxytocin.
- These hormones are associated with pleasure, mood regulation, and social bonding.

• **Stress Reduction**:

- Music can lower levels of cortisol, the stress hormone.
- This can help reduce anxiety and agitation common in dementia.

• **Emotional Memory Activation**:

- Familiar music can evoke emotional memories, even when other memories have faded.
- This can provide a sense of connection to one's past and identity.

Choosing Uplifting and Mood-Boosting Songs

Selecting the right music is crucial for maximizing its emotional benefits. Here are some tips for choosing mood-boosting songs:

1. **Focus on Personal Preferences**:
    - Choose music from your loved one's young adult years (ages 18-25).
    - Consider their cultural background and musical tastes.
2. **Opt for Positive Lyrics and Melodies**:
    - Select songs with uplifting messages and cheerful tunes.
    - Avoid songs with potentially upsetting lyrics or themes.
3. **Consider Tempo and Rhythm**:

- For energy and mood elevation, choose songs with a moderate to upbeat tempo.
- For relaxation, opt for slower, gentler rhythms.

4. **Create Themed Playlists**:
   - Develop playlists for different moods or times of day.
   - Examples: "Morning Energy," "Relaxing Afternoon," "Bedtime Calm"

Here's a table with examples of mood-boosting songs from different eras:

Era	Uplifting Song Examples
1940s-1950s	"Singin' in the Rain" - Gene Kelly "What a Wonderful World" - Louis Armstrong
1960s-1970s	"Here Comes the Sun" - The Beatles "Dancing Queen" - ABBA
1980s-1990s	"Don't Stop Believin'" - Journey "Walking on Sunshine" - Katrina and The Waves

Addressing Depression and Apathy Through Music

Music therapy can be a powerful tool in combating depression and apathy, which are common challenges in dementia:

• **Structured Music Sessions**:

- Regular, scheduled music activities can provide a sense of routine and purpose.
- This can help combat feelings of apathy and disengagement.

• **Active Participation**:

- Encourage singing, clapping, or moving to the music.
- Physical engagement can boost mood and energy levels.

• **Social Connection**:

- Group music activities can foster a sense of belonging and social interaction.
- This can help alleviate feelings of isolation and depression.

- **Personalized Playlists for Emotional Support**:
  - Create playlists specifically designed to lift mood during difficult times.
  - Include songs that have personal significance or evoke positive memories.

- **Combining Music with Other Activities**:
  - Incorporate music into daily routines like bathing or dressing.
  - This can make potentially stressful activities more enjoyable and reduce resistance.

Remember, the impact of music can vary from person to person and even day to day. Be patient and observant; don't be afraid to experiment with different music and activities. Your efforts to bring music into your loved one's life can significantly impact their emotional well-being and quality of life.

By understanding and harnessing the power of music, you're providing a valuable gift to your loved one with dementia. Music can offer moments of joy, connection, and emotional expression, even as other forms of communication become challenging. Your dedication to enhancing your loved one's mood and emotional well-being through music is commendable.

Improving Social Interaction and Communication

As a caregiver or family member of someone with dementia, you've likely witnessed how challenging social interaction and communication can become. Music therapy offers a powerful way to bridge these gaps, creating opportunities for connection and expression. Let's explore how music can enhance social interaction and communication for your loved one with dementia.

Group Music Activities for Socialization

Group music activities provide a structured, enjoyable way for people with dementia to interact with others. These activities can:

• **Reduce feelings of isolation**: Group settings allow participants to feel part of a community.

• **Encourage participation**: Even those hesitant to speak can join in by clapping, tapping their feet, or humming.

• **Promote turn-taking and cooperation**: Activities like passing instruments or taking turns leading a song help reinforce social skills.

• **Create shared experiences**: Participating in music together builds a sense of camaraderie and shared accomplishment.

Here are some examples of group music activities that can enhance socialization:

1. **Sing-alongs**: Familiar songs encourage participation and reminiscence.
2. **Rhythm circles**: Using simple percussion instruments to create rhythms together.
3. **Musical bingo**: Combining a familiar game with music recognition.
4. **Movement to music**: Simple dance or exercise routines set to music.

Using Music to Facilitate Non-Verbal Communication

For many people with dementia, verbal communication becomes increasingly difficult. Music can provide alternative ways to express emotions and connect with others:

• **Emotional expression**: Music can help individuals express feelings they may struggle to express.

• **Rhythmic communication**: Matching rhythms with another person can create a sense of connection and understanding.

• **Facial expressions and body language**: Observing reactions to music can provide insights into a person's mood or preferences.

• **Musical choices**: Selecting songs or instruments can allow individuals to express their personality and preferences.

Table: Non-Verbal Communication Through Music

Musical Element	Potential Communication
Tempo	Energy level or mood
Volume	Intensity of emotion
Instrument choice	Personal preference or past experiences
Lyrics (even if not sung)	Thoughts or memories

Strengthening Family Bonds Through Shared Musical Experiences

Music can be a powerful tool for maintaining and strengthening connections between individuals with dementia and their family members:

1. **Creating new memories**: Engaging in music can create positive, new experiences to cherish.
2. **Connecting to the past**: Sharing favorite songs from the past can evoke memories and spark conversations.
3. **Expressing affection**: Singing or dancing together can be a way to show love and care non-verbally.
4. **Reducing caregiver stress**: Shared musical experiences can be enjoyable for the person with dementia and their caregiver, providing a break from routine care tasks.

Tips for incorporating music into family interactions:

• **Create a family playlist**: Compile songs that are meaningful to your family history.

• **Have regular music sessions**: Set aside time each week for a family "concert" or sing-along.

• **Use music during care routines**: Incorporate favorite songs into daily activities like dressing or meal times.

• **Attend concerts together**: Look for dementia-friendly musical events in your community.

Remember, the goal is not musical perfection but rather connection and enjoyment. Even if your loved one can't actively participate in making music, simply listening together can be a powerful bonding experience.

By incorporating music into social interactions and family time, you're providing entertainment and opportunities for meaningful connection, expression, and joy. Your efforts to use music as a bridge to communication can significantly enhance your loved one's quality of life and strengthen your relationship, even as dementia progresses.

Finding and Working with a Certified Music Therapist

As a caregiver or family member of someone with dementia, you may be considering professional music therapy to enhance your loved one's care. Working with a certified music therapist can provide structured, evidence-based interventions tailored to your loved one's specific needs. Let's explore how to find and work with a qualified music therapist.

Qualifications to Look For

When seeking a music therapist, it's vital to ensure they have the proper qualifications and experience to work with dementia patients.

Educational Requirements for Music Therapists

• **Bachelor's Degree (minimum)**: In music therapy or a related field
• **Master's or Doctoral Degree**: Often preferred, especially for specialized work
• **Clinical Training**: Completion of a supervised clinical internship

Certifications and Specializations in Dementia Care

1. **Board Certification**: Look for the designation MT-BC (Music Therapist-Board Certified)
2. **Neurologic Music Therapy (NMT)**: Specialized training in using music for neurological conditions
3. **Dementia Care Certification**: Additional training specific to working with dementia patients

Experience and Skills to Consider

- **Years of Practice**: Preferably with experience in geriatric care or dementia
- **Communication Skills**: Ability to interact effectively with patients and families
- **Adaptability**: Skill in modifying interventions based on patient needs
- **Empathy and Patience**: Essential qualities for working with dementia patients

How to Find a Local Music Therapist

Finding a qualified music therapist in your area can be done through various channels:

Professional Associations and Directories

- **American Music Therapy Association (AMTA)**: Offers a "Find a Music Therapist" directory
- **Certification Board for Music Therapists (CBMT)**: Provides a searchable database of certified therapists

Referrals from Healthcare Providers

- Ask your loved one's physician, neurologist, or geriatrician for recommendations
- Inquire at local hospitals or memory care facilities about music therapy services

Online Resources and Databases

- **Local Alzheimer's Association Chapter**: You may have information on music therapists in your area
- **Senior Care Directories**: Often include listings for various therapy services, including music therapy

Questions to Ask When Hiring a Music Therapist

When interviewing potential music therapists, consider asking the following questions:

Assessment Process and Treatment Planning

- "How do you assess a patient's needs and preferences?"
- "How do you develop and adjust treatment plans?"
- "What specific techniques do you use for dementia patients?"

Frequency and Duration of Sessions

- "How often do you recommend sessions?"
- "How long does a typical session last?"
- "Do you offer both individual and group sessions?"

Costs and Insurance Coverage

- "What are your fees for individual and group sessions?"
- "Do you offer any sliding scale or payment plans?"
- "Can you assist with insurance claims for music therapy?"

What to Expect During a Music Therapy Session

Understanding the structure and goals of music therapy sessions can help you prepare and make the most of this intervention.

Typical Session Structure and Activities

Phase	Activities	Duration
Opening	Greetings, orientation to time/place	5-10 minutes
Active Music Making	Singing, instrument play, movement	20-30 minutes
Receptive Listening	Guided relaxation, reminiscence	10-15 minutes
Closure	Summary, goodbye song	5-10 minutes

Involvement of Family Members and Caregivers

- **Observation**: You may be invited to watch and learn techniques
- **Participation**: Some therapists encourage family involvement in sessions
- **Home Practice**: The therapist may suggest activities to do between sessions

Goal-Setting and Progress Evaluation

- **Initial Goals**: Often focus on mood, cognitive stimulation, and social engagement
- **Regular Assessments**: Therapists typically evaluate progress every few sessions
- **Adjustments**: Treatment plans are modified based on response and changing needs

Remember, finding the right music therapist is a process. Don't hesitate to ask questions and express your concerns. A good therapist will happily explain their approach and work with you to ensure the best care for your loved one.

By finding a qualified music therapist and understanding what to expect, you're taking an essential step in enhancing your loved one's care. Music therapy can offer unique benefits for individuals with dementia, potentially improving their quality of life and providing moments of joy and connection. Your dedication to exploring this option is commendable and reflects the depth of your care and commitment.

Do-it-yourself (DIY) Music Interventions: Bringing Music Therapy Home

As a caregiver or family member of someone with dementia, you play a crucial role in enhancing your loved one's quality of life. While professional music therapy can be beneficial, you can also bring the power of music into your home with do-it-yourself interventions. Let's explore how to create personalized playlists that can provide comfort, stimulation, and joy for your loved one with dementia.

Creating a Personalized Playlist

A well-crafted playlist can be a powerful tool in dementia care, offering familiar comfort and stimulating memories. Here's how to create an influential personalized playlist:

Identifying Meaningful Songs from Different Life Stages

1. **Early Years (Childhood to Young Adulthood)**:

   • Nursery rhymes and children's songs
   • Popular music from their teenage years
   • Songs associated with school or college experiences

2. **Young Adult Years (18-25)**:

   • Wedding songs or music from significant relationships
   • Popular hits from this era (often the most emotionally impactful)
   • Music related to their career or significant life events

3. **Middle Adulthood**:
   • Songs associated with their children's childhood
   • Music from family vacations or special occasions
   • Work-related songs or music from their professional life

4. **Later Years**:
   • Songs enjoyed with grandchildren
   • Music from hobbies or retirement activities
   • Spiritual or religious music, if relevant

Tips for Identifying Meaningful Songs:

- Ask family members and friends for input
- Look through old photos or home videos for musical clues
- Consider cultural and ethnic background when selecting music

Balancing Familiar and New Music

Creating an influential playlist involves striking a balance between familiar comfort and novel stimulation:

Familiar Music	New Music
Provides comfort and security	Offers cognitive stimulation
Triggers memories and emotions	Prevents boredom and maintains interest
It helps manage anxiety and agitation.	Can introduce new positive experiences

Guidelines for Balancing:

- Aim for about 70-80% familiar music and 20-30% new music
- Introduce new music gradually, observing reactions
- Choose new music that's similar in style or era to familiar favorites

Tools and Apps for Playlist Creation

Several tools and apps can help you create and manage personalized playlists:

1. **Spotify**:
    - Offers a vast library of music
    - Allows creation of collaborative playlists for family input
    - Provides "Discover Weekly" for new music suggestions
2. **Apple Music**:
    - Integrates seamlessly with Apple devices
    - Offers curated playlists and personalized recommendations
    - Allows easy sharing of playlists among family members
3. **Vera**:
    - Specifically designed for people with dementia
    - Creates AI-generated playlists based on birth year and preferences
    - Offers different playlists for various moods and times of day
4. **MindMate**:
    - Combines music with other cognitive stimulation activities
    - Provides brain games and exercises alongside music
    - Offers nutritional and physical exercise advice

5. **YouTube**:
    - Free platform with a vast array of music
    - Allows creation of playlists with both audio and video content
    - Offers the ability to find rare or obscure songs

Tips for Using Music Apps:

- Ensure the app is easy to navigate for both you and your loved one
- Look for apps that allow offline playback for areas with poor internet
- Consider apps that integrate with smart speakers for hands-free use

Remember, creating a personalized playlist is an ongoing process. Be patient and observant, noting which songs elicit positive responses and which might cause distress. Don't be afraid to adjust the playlist as your loved one's preferences or needs change.

Creating thoughtful, personalized playlists provides more than entertainment—you're offering a powerful tool for emotional regulation, cognitive stimulation, and connection. Your efforts in bringing music into your loved one's daily life can significantly improve their well-being and quality of life.

Choosing the Right Equipment for Music Playback

As a caregiver or family member of a senior with dementia, selecting the appropriate music playback equipment is crucial for creating a positive and engaging music experience at home. Let's explore how to choose user-friendly devices, compare headphones and speakers, and consider adaptive equipment for hearing impairments.

Selecting User-Friendly Devices for Seniors

When choosing a music playback device for seniors, especially those with dementia, simplicity and ease of use are key. Here are some factors to consider:

1. **Simple Controls**: Look for devices with large, clearly labeled buttons for essential functions like play, pause, and volume control.

2. **Limited Features**: Avoid devices with complex menus or multiple functions that may confuse the user.
3. **Durability**: Choose devices that can withstand accidental drops or spills.
4. **Battery Life**: Opt for devices with long or easy-to-use charging systems.
5. **Familiarity**: Consider devices that resemble familiar objects, like traditional radios or record players.

Recommended User-Friendly Devices:

- Simple MP3 players with large buttons
- One-touch music players designed for seniors
- Smart speakers with voice control (if appropriate for the user)
- Retro-style radios with modern internals

Headphones vs. Speakers: Pros and Cons

Both headphones and speakers have advantages and disadvantages regarding music playback for seniors with dementia. Let's compare:

Aspect	Headphones	Speakers
Sound Isolation	Better to focus on music	Allow awareness of surroundings
Comfort	It may be uncomfortable for long periods	No physical contact is required
Mobility	Restrict movement	Allow free movement
Social Aspect	Individual experience	Can be shared with others
Volume Control	Easier to manage for individual	May disturb others if too loud
Hygiene	Require regular cleaning	Less maintenance needed

Pros of Headphones:

- Provide a more immersive experience
- Can be used in shared spaces without disturbing others
- Often offer better sound quality at lower volumes

Cons of Headphones:

- May be confusing or uncomfortable for some seniors
- Can isolate the user from their environment
- Potential safety risk if the user can't hear essential sounds

Pros of Speakers:
• Allow for a shared music experience
• No need to wear anything
• Can fill a room with sound, creating ambiance

Cons of Speakers:
• May disturb others in shared living spaces
• Sound quality can be affected by room acoustics
• Harder to control volume for individual needs

Adaptive Equipment for Hearing Impairments

For seniors with hearing impairments, adaptive equipment can enhance the music listening experience:

1. **Amplified Headphones**: These provide an extra volume boost and can be helpful for those with mild to moderate hearing loss.
2. **Bone Conduction Headphones**: These bypass the outer ear and may benefit certain types of hearing loss.
3. **Wireless TV Listeners**: These devices can connect to TVs or other audio sources and transmit sound directly to headphones or hearing aids.
4. **Hearing Aid Compatible Devices**: Look for music players compatible with hearing aids' telecoil function.
5. **Vibrating Pillows or Wearables**: These can add a tactile element to the music experience for those with severe hearing loss.

Tips for Adapting Equipment:

• **Consult an Audiologist**: They can recommend specific devices based on the individual's hearing needs.
• **Start Simple**: Begin with essential adaptive equipment and gradually introduce more complex options if needed.
• **Consider Comfort**: Ensure any wearable devices are comfortable for long-term use.
• **Regular Maintenance**: Keep adaptive equipment clean and well-maintained for optimal performance.

Remember, the best equipment is the one your loved one will use and enjoy. Finding the perfect setup may take some trial and error, but the benefits of bringing music into their daily life are well worth the effort.

Don't hesitate to consult healthcare professionals or music therapists for personalized recommendations.

By thoughtfully selecting and adapting music playback equipment, you're creating opportunities for your loved one to engage with music in a way that's comfortable and enjoyable for them. This can improve mood, cognitive stimulation, and overall quality of life.

Incorporating Singing and Instrument Play

As a caregiver or family member of someone with dementia, you can bring the joy and benefits of active music-making into your loved one's daily life. Singing and playing simple instruments can provide cognitive stimulation, emotional expression, and physical engagement. Let's explore how you can incorporate these activities at home.

Simple Instruments for Home Use

Introducing easy-to-use instruments can make music-making accessible and enjoyable for your loved one. Here are some instruments well-suited for home use:

1. **Percussion Instruments**:
   - Tambourine
   - Maracas or egg shakers
   - Hand drums (e.g., djembe or bongo)
   - Rhythm sticks
2. **Melodic Instruments**:
   - Xylophone or glockenspiel
   - Kalimba (thumb piano)
   - Harmonica
3. **Adaptive Instruments**:
   - Boomwhackers (color-coded tuned percussion tubes)
   - Adaptive guitar or ukulele (with simplified chord buttons)

Tips for Choosing Instruments:

- Select instruments that are lightweight and easy to hold
- Opt for instruments that produce sound with minimal effort
- Consider instruments that relate to your loved one's past musical experiences

Benefits of Singing, Even for Non-Musicians

Singing is a natural and accessible form of music-making that offers numerous benefits, regardless of musical ability:

Benefit	Description
Cognitive Stimulation	Engages memory, attention, and language processing
Emotional Expression	Provides an outlet for expressing and regulating emotions
Social Connection	Creates opportunities for bonding and shared experiences
Physical Exercise	It supports breath control and can improve posture.
Mood Enhancement	Releases endorphins and can reduce stress and anxiety

Encouraging Singing at Home:

1. **Start with Familiar Songs**: Choose well-known tunes from your loved one's past.
2. **Use Lyric Sheets**: Provide large-print lyrics to support participation.
3. **Sing During Daily Activities**: Incorporate songs into routines like bathing or dressing.
4. **Create a Judgment-Free Zone**: Emphasize enjoyment over perfection.
5. **Join In** Sing to show that everyone can participate, regardless of ability.

Rhythm Exercises for Motor Skills

Engaging in rhythmic activities can help maintain and improve motor skills, coordination, and cognitive function. Here are some simple exercises you can try:

1. **Basic Beat Keeping**:

    • Clap or tap along to the beat of a familiar song
    • Use rhythm sticks or drums to maintain a steady beat

2. **Call and Response**:

    • Create a simple rhythm and have your loved one repeat it back
    • Gradually increase complexity as abilities allow

3. **Body Percussion**:

    • Combine claps, pats, and stomps to create rhythmic patterns
    • Follow along with instructional videos for more structured activities

4. **Rhythm and Movement**:

    • Incorporate simple dance moves with rhythmic patterns
    • Use scarves or ribbons to add visual interest to movements

Rhythm Exercise Progression:

1. Start with slow, simple rhythms
2. Gradually increase the tempo as comfort and ability improve
3. Introduce syncopation or more complex patterns over time
4. Combine rhythm exercises with familiar songs

Remember, the goal is engagement and enjoyment, not perfection. Celebrate any level of participation and be patient as your loved one explores these activities.

Tips for Successful Music-Making Sessions:

• **Keep Sessions Short**: Start with 10-15 minute sessions and extend as interest allows
• **Follow Their Lead**: Pay attention to your loved one's energy and engagement levels
• **Be Flexible**: Be ready to switch activities if one isn't resonating
• **Make It Routine**: Try to incorporate music-making at consistent times each day
• **Stay Positive**: Offer encouragement and focus on the joy of making music together.

By incorporating singing and instrument play into your caregiving routine, you're providing more than just entertainment. You're offering opportunities for cognitive stimulation, emotional expression, and physical engagement. These activities can create joy, connection, and accomplishment for you and your loved one.

Remember, you don't need to be a trained musician to bring music into your home. What matters most is your willingness to explore and engage in these activities with your loved one. Your efforts in creating a musical environment can significantly enhance their quality of life and provide meaningful shared experiences.

Using Music for Daily Activities and Routines

As a caregiver or family member of someone with dementia, you've likely noticed how challenging daily activities and routines can become. Music can be a powerful tool to enhance these everyday moments, creating a more positive and engaging environment for your loved one. Let's explore how you can incorporate music into daily activities and routines to improve the caregiving experience for both you and your loved one.

Background Music for Meals and Personal Care

Using background music during meals and personal care activities can create a calming atmosphere and potentially improve your loved one's cooperation and enjoyment of these essential daily tasks.

Benefits of background music during meals:

• Reduces anxiety and agitation
• Encourages appetite and food intake
• Creates a pleasant social atmosphere
• Masks potentially distracting noises

Tips for using music during meals:

1. Choose familiar, upbeat music with a moderate tempo
2. Keep the volume at a comfortable level that allows for conversation
3. Avoid music with complex lyrics that might be distracting
4. Consider creating a specific "mealtime playlist" to establish a routine

Benefits of background music during personal care:

- Reduces stress and anxiety during potentially uncomfortable tasks
- Provides distraction from discomfort or embarrassment
- Can improve cooperation with caregiving tasks
- Creates a more pleasant experience for both caregiver and care recipient

Tips for using music during personal care:

1. Select calming, soothing music for potentially stressful activities like bathing
2. Use upbeat, energizing music for morning routines to help with waking up
3. Sing along to familiar songs to engage your loved one and create a positive atmosphere
4. Be prepared to adjust or turn off the music if it becomes overstimulating

Musical Cues for Transitions and Tasks

Music can be a powerful cue to signal transitions between activities or prompt specific tasks. This can be especially helpful for individuals with dementia who struggle with time awareness or task initiation.

Examples of musical cues:

Activity/Transition	Musical Cue
Waking up	Gentle, gradually increasing tempo
Mealtime	Familiar dinner music or food-related songs
Medication time	Short, catchy jingle or specific song snippet
Bedtime routine	Slow, calming lullaby or relaxation music

Implementing musical cues:

1. **Choose distinctive music**: Select music easily recognizable and associated with the specific activity or transition.
2. **Be consistent**: Establish a routine using the same musical cue for each daily activity.
3. **Gradually introduce**: Start by playing the music while verbally explaining the associated task, then gradually reduce verbal prompts as the association strengthens.

4. **Keep it brief**: Musical cues should be short (30 seconds to 2 minutes) to avoid overstimulation.
5. **Observe and adjust**: Pay attention to your loved one's reactions and be prepared to modify the cues if they're ineffective.

Creating a Soundtrack for the Day

Developing a "soundtrack" for your loved one's day can provide structure, stimulation, and emotional support throughout their daily routine.

Steps to create a daily soundtrack:

1. **Map out the day**: List the main activities and transitions in your loved one's typical day.
2. **Match music to activities**: Select appropriate music for each part of the day, considering tempo, mood, and familiarity.
3. **Create playlists**: Organize the selected music into playlists for different times of day or activities.
4. **Be flexible**: Allow spontaneity and changes based on your loved one's mood and needs.

Sample daily soundtrack structure:

• **Morning wake-up**: Gentle, gradually more upbeat music
• **Breakfast and morning routine**: Cheerful, familiar tunes
• **Mid-morning activities**: Stimulating music for engagement
• **Lunchtime**: Calm, pleasant background music
• **Afternoon rest**: Soft, soothing melodies
• **Late afternoon activities**: Moderately upbeat, familiar songs
• **Dinner and evening routine**: Relaxing, comforting music
• **Bedtime**: Very slow, calming lullabies or nature sounds

Tips for implementing a daily soundtrack:

• Use a music player with a timer function to automatically transition between playlists
• Keep the overall volume at a comfortable level throughout the day
• Be prepared to adjust or turn off music if it becomes overwhelming
• Include periods of silence to prevent overstimulation
• Regularly review and update the soundtrack based on your loved one's responses

Remember, using music in daily activities and routines aims to enhance your loved one's quality of life and ease the caregiving process. Be patient and observant as you implement these strategies, and don't hesitate to adjust your approach based on your loved one's reactions. Your efforts to create a musically enriched environment can lead to more positive interactions, improved mood, and a greater connection between you and your loved one with dementia.

Implementing a Music Program in Your Dementia Care Routine

Establishing a Regular Music Schedule

As a caregiver or family member of someone with dementia, incorporating a consistent music program into your care routine can provide structure, comfort, and cognitive stimulation for your loved one. Let's explore how to create a balanced and effective music schedule that enhances your caregiving experience.

Integrating Music into Daily and Weekly Routines

Creating a regular music schedule helps establish a sense of familiarity and can aid in managing the symptoms of dementia. Here's how you can integrate music into your daily and weekly routines:

Daily Music Integration:

1. **Morning Wake-Up**: Start the day with gentle, uplifting music to ease the transition from sleep to wakefulness.
2. **Meal Times**: Play soft background music during breakfast, lunch, and dinner to create a pleasant atmosphere and potentially improve appetite.
3. **Activity Periods**: Use more stimulating music during exercise or cognitive activities to enhance engagement.
4. **Rest Periods**: Incorporate calming music during quiet times or naps to promote relaxation.
5. **Evening Wind-Down**: End the day with soothing melodies to signal bedtime and aid in relaxation.

Weekly Music Activities:

- **Monday**: Group sing-along session
- **Wednesday**: Music and movement exercise
- **Friday**: Music listening and reminiscence activity
- **Sunday**: Relaxation and meditation with music

Sample Daily Music Schedule:

Time	Activity	Music Type
7:00 AM	Wake-Up	Gentle, gradually upbeat
8:00 AM	Breakfast	Soft, familiar tunes
10:00 AM	Morning Activity	Stimulating, rhythmic
12:00 PM	Lunch	Calm background music
2:00 PM	Rest Period	Soft, instrumental
4:00 PM	Afternoon Activity	Upbeat, engaging
6:00 PM	Dinner	Pleasant, familiar melodies
8:00 PM	Evening Wind-Down	Slow, soothing music

Balancing Structured Sessions with Spontaneous Music Use

While a structured music schedule is beneficial, allowing for spontaneous musical moments is equally essential. This balance can help maintain interest and address immediate emotional or behavioral needs.

Structured Sessions:

- Planned daily music activities (e.g., morning sing-along)
- Weekly group music events
- Scheduled music therapy sessions (if applicable)**Spontaneous Music Use:**
- Playing a favorite song when your loved one seems anxious
- Impromptu dance sessions during moments of high-energy
- Humming or singing during care activities as needed

Tips for Maintaining Balance:

1. **Be Flexible**: Allow your structured schedule to bend when necessary to accommodate your loved one's changing needs or moods.
2. **Keep Music Accessible**: Have a music player and a variety of playlists readily available for spontaneous use.

3. **Observe and Respond**: Listen to your loved one's cues and use music responsively throughout the day.
4. **Involve Others**: Encourage family members or other caregivers to engage in structured and spontaneous music activities.

Tracking Responses and Adjusting the Schedule

To ensure your music program remains effective, it's crucial to monitor your loved one's responses and make adjustments as needed.

Creating a Music Response Log:

Date	Time	Music/Activity	Mood Before	Mood After	Notes
5/1	10 AM	Sing-along	Agitated	Calm	They enjoyed "You Are My Sunshine."
5/2	2 PM	Classical Listening	Lethargic	Alert	Tapped foot to rhythm
5/3	7 PM	Bedtime playlist	Restless	Sleepy	Fell asleep after 15 min

Tips for Effective Tracking and Adjusting:

1. **Be Consistent**: Try to log responses daily, even if briefly.
2. **Look for Patterns**: Notice if certain music or activities consistently produce positive responses.
3. **Involve Your Loved One**: Ask for their feedback on the music and activities if possible.
4. **Be Patient**: Give new additions to the schedule at least a week before deciding if they're effective.
5. **Regularly Review**: Set aside time each month to review your logs and adjust the music schedule.
6. **Consult Professionals**: Share your observations with healthcare providers or a music therapist for additional insights and recommendations.

Remember, implementing a music program aims to enhance your loved one's quality of life and ease the caregiving process. Be patient with yourself and your loved one as you establish this new routine. Celebrate small victories, such as a smile during a favorite song or a moment of calm during a previously tricky time of day.

Your dedication to creating a nurturing, music-filled environment for your loved one with dementia is admirable. Establishing a regular music schedule, balancing structure with spontaneity, and carefully tracking responses provide a valuable source of comfort, stimulation, and connection. Your efforts can make a significant difference in managing the challenges of dementia and creating moments of joy in your daily caregiving journey.

Adapting Music Interventions to Different Stages of Dementia

As a caregiver or family member of someone with dementia, you understand that the condition progresses over time, affecting your loved one's abilities and needs. It's crucial to adapt your music interventions to match these changing requirements. Let's explore how to tailor your music program for each stage of dementia, ensuring that your loved one receives the most benefit and enjoyment possible.

Early-Stage: Focus on Active Participation and Learning

In the early stages of dementia, your loved one may retain many cognitive abilities and actively engage in music activities. This is an excellent time to introduce new musical experiences and build on existing skills.

Key Objectives:

- Maintain cognitive function
- Encourage social interaction
- Build confidence and self-esteem
- Create new positive experiences

Suggested Activities:

1. **Group Sing-Alongs**: Organize regular singing sessions with family and friends.
2. **Music Lessons**: If interested, encourage learning or continuing to play an instrument.
3. **Music Appreciation Classes**: Attend or create sessions to explore different genres and composers.
4. **Rhythm Games**: Introduce games that challenge memory and coordination through rhythm.
5. **Music-Based Exercise**: Participate in dance classes or movement activities set to music.

Tips for Early-Stage Music Interventions:

- Encourage active participation and decision-making in music choices
- Introduce a variety of music styles to maintain interest and cognitive engagement
- Use music as a tool for reminiscence and life review
- Create opportunities for social interaction through music events or groups

Middle-Stage: Emphasizing Familiar Music and Emotional Connection

As dementia progresses to the middle stage, your loved one may experience increased confusion and difficulty with complex tasks. At this stage, familiar music becomes increasingly essential for creating a sense of security and evoking memories.

Key Objectives:

- Provide emotional comfort and reduce anxiety
- Maintain a connection to personal identity and memories
- Manage behavioral symptoms
- Support daily routines

Suggested Activities:

1. **Personalized Playlists**: Create playlists of favorite songs from your loved one's young adult years.
2. **Music and Movement**: Encourage simple dance movements or seated exercises to familiar tunes.
3. **Sing-Alongs with Lyric Sheets**: Provide large-print lyrics to support participation in singing.
4. **Music-Assisted ADLs**: Incorporate familiar songs into daily activities like dressing or bathing.
5. **Rhythm Activities**: Use simple percussion instruments for engaging rhythm exercises.

Tips for Middle-Stage Music Interventions:

• Focus on music from your loved one's young adult years (ages 18-25)
• Use music to create a calm environment during potentially stressful activities
• Encourage participation, but don't pressure if your loved one prefers to listen
• Be prepared to adapt activities based on daily fluctuations in ability and mood

Late-Stage: Using Music for Comfort and Sensory Stimulation

In the late stages of dementia, the focus shifts to providing comfort, managing pain, and offering sensory stimulation through music. Even when other forms of communication become difficult, music can often still reach and soothe your loved one.

Key Objectives:

• Provide sensory stimulation
• Offer comfort and pain management
• Maintain connection and quality of life
• Support end-of-life care

Suggested Activities:

1. **Gentle Music Listening**: Play soft, soothing music, particularly during rest times or medical procedures.
2. **Singing or Humming**: Offer close, personal interaction by singing or humming familiar tunes.
3. **Rhythmic Touch**: Combine gentle touch or massage with rhythmic music.
4. **Music and Aromatherapy**: Pair calming scents with soothing music for multi-sensory comfort.
5. **Personalized Lullabies**: Use familiar, gentle songs to aid sleep or relaxation.

Tips for Late-Stage Music Interventions:

• Pay close attention to non-verbal cues to gauge comfort and preferences
• Use headphones if your loved one is sensitive to environmental noise
• Incorporate music into pain management strategies in consultation with healthcare providers
• Continue to use music as a way to connect, even if your loved one seems unresponsive

Table: Music Interventions Across Dementia Stages

Stage	Focus	Key Activities	Considerations
Early	Active participation & learning	Group sing-alongs, music lessons, appreciation classes	Encourage choice and variety
Middle	Familiar music & emotional connection	Personalized playlists, music-assisted ADLs, simple rhythm activities	Focus on comfort and routine
Late	Comfort & sensory stimulation	Gentle listening, singing/humming, rhythmic touch	Prioritize soothing and familiar sounds

Remember, these stages are general guidelines, and your loved one's experience with dementia is unique. Be prepared to adjust your approach based on their individual needs and responses. The most important thing is to continue using music for connection, comfort, and improved quality of life throughout their journey with dementia.

Your dedication to adapting and maintaining a music program for your loved one is admirable. By tailoring your music interventions to each stage of dementia, you're providing a valuable source of comfort, stimulation, and connection. Your efforts can make a significant difference in managing the challenges of dementia and creating moments of joy, even in the later stages of the condition.

Combining Music with Other Activities

As a caregiver or family member of someone with dementia, you've likely discovered the power of music in enhancing your loved one's quality of life. But did you know combining music with other activities can amplify its benefits? Let's explore how you can integrate music with movement, art, and storytelling to create engaging and meaningful experiences for your loved one.

Music and Movement Exercises

Combining music with physical movement can provide cognitive and physical benefits for individuals with dementia. Here are some ways to incorporate music and movement:

1. **Chair Exercises**: Use upbeat music to accompany simple seated exercises.

    • Arm raises
    • Leg lifts
    • Gentle twists

2. **Dance Sessions**: Encourage your loved one to move to the rhythm, standing or seated.

    • Slow waltzes for balance
    • Hand jives for coordination
    • Swaying to ballads for relaxation

3. **Rhythm and Motion**: Using percussion instruments to create moving rhythms.

    • Marching in place while shaking maracas
    • Tapping feet while playing hand drums
    • Clapping along to familiar tunes

Benefits of Music and Movement:

- Improves circulation and flexibility
- Enhances mood and reduces anxiety
- Promotes social interaction
- Stimulates cognitive function through multi-tasking

Table: Sample Music and Movement Session

Time	Activity	Music Type	Benefits
5 min	Warm-up stretches	Slow, calming melodies	Gentle awakening of the body
10 min	Seated dance moves	Upbeat, familiar songs	Cardiovascular exercise, memory stimulation
10 min	Rhythm with instruments	Songs with strong beats	Hand-eye coordination, cognitive engagement
5 min	Cool-down and relaxation	Soft, soothing music	Stress reduction, transition to next activity

Art and Crafts with Musical Themes

Combining music with art activities can stimulate creativity and evoke memories. Here are some ideas:

• **Painting to Music**: Play different genres of music and encourage painting based on the emotions or memories the music evokes

.• **Musical Instrument Crafts**: Create simple instruments like shakers or drums using household items, then play along to favorite songs.

• **Album Cover Collages**: Use old album covers or printed images to create collages, discussing memories associated with the music.

• **Musical Note Art**: Draw or paint extensive musical notes, filling them with colors or patterns inspired by different songs.

Tips for Music-Inspired Art Sessions:

1. Choose music that your loved one enjoys and finds familiar.
2. Keep art supplies simple and safe (e.g., non-toxic paints, safety scissors).
3. Focus on the process rather than the result.
4. Display finished artwork to boost self-esteem and spark conversations.

Storytelling and Reminiscence Through Songs

Music can be a powerful tool for evoking memories and encouraging storytelling. Here's how you can use songs to stimulate reminiscence:

1. **Song Lyric Prompts**:
    - Choose songs with meaningful lyrics
    - Read or sing a line, then pause to ask about related memories
    - Example: "When I'm 64" by The Beatles can prompt discussions about aging, family, or past relationships
2. **Era-Based Playlists**:
    - Create playlists from different decades of your loved one's life
    - Play songs and encourage sharing of memories from that time
    - Discuss historical events, fashion, or personal experiences related to the music
3. **Personal History Soundtrack**:
    - Compile songs that represent different stages of your loved one's life
    - Use these as prompts to create a musical biography
    - Encourage storytelling about why each song is significant
4. **Musical Photo Albums**:
    - Pair family photos with songs from the same period
    - Look through the album together, playing the associated songs
    - Ask open-ended questions about the memories in the photos and how the music relates

Benefits of Musical Reminiscence:

- Stimulates long-term memory
- Encourages verbal communication
- Provides emotional comfort through familiar songs
- Creates opportunities for sharing and connection

Remember, these activities aim to create enjoyable, meaningful experiences for your loved one with dementia. Be patient, flexible, and ready to adapt activities based on their responses and energy levels. Celebrate small moments of engagement and connection, as these can be profoundly impactful for both you and your loved one.

Combining music with movement, art, and storytelling creates multi-sensory experiences that can enhance cognitive function, improve mood, and provide opportunities for self-expression and social connection. Your efforts to enrich your loved one's life through these creative activities are commendable and can make a significant difference in their daily experience with dementia.

Monitoring and Adjusting Your Approach

As a dedicated caregiver or family member of someone with dementia, you've incorporated music into your care routine. Monitoring its impact and making adjustments as needed regularly is crucial to ensuring that your music program remains effective and beneficial. Let's explore how you can observe responses, journal, and collaborate with healthcare providers to optimize your music interventions.

Observing Verbal and Non-Verbal Responses to Music

People with dementia may not always be able to express their feelings about music verbally, so paying attention to verbal and non-verbal cues is essential. Here's what to look for:

Verbal Responses:

- Singing or humming along
- Commenting on the music
- Sharing memories triggered by songs
- Requesting specific songs or artists

Non-Verbal Responses:

- Facial expressions (smiling, frowning)
- Body language (relaxing, tensing up)
- Movement (tapping feet, clapping hands)
- Changes in breathing patterns

Table: Common Responses to Music and Their Potential Meanings

Response	Potential Meaning
Smiling, relaxed posture	Enjoyment, comfort
Agitation, trying to leave	Overstimulation, dislike of music
Increased alertness	Cognitive engagement
Tearfulness	Emotional connection, possibly bittersweet memories
Physical movement	Rhythm engagement, desire to participate

Tips for Effective Observation:

1. **Be Present**: Give your full attention during music sessions to notice subtle responses.
2. **Start Simple**: Begin with clear, easily observable reactions before looking for more nuanced responses.
3. **Consider Context**: When observing responses, note the time of day, the environment, and your loved one's general mood.
4. **Be Patient**: Some responses may be delayed or subtle, especially in the later stages of dementia.
5. **Involve Others**: Ask other caregivers or family members to share their observations.

Keeping a Music Therapy Journal

Maintaining a journal can help you track the effectiveness of your music program over time and identify patterns or preferences. Here's how to create and use a music therapy journal:

What to Include in Your Journal:

- Date and time of music session
- Songs or types of music played
- Duration of the session

- Your loved one's mood before and after
- Specific responses observed
- Any notable events or changes in routine that day

Sample Journal Entry Format:

Entry	Details
Date:	
Time:	
Music Played [Song titles or genre]	
Duration [Length of the session]	
Mood before:	
Mood after:	
Responses Observed	
Notes	

Tips for Effective Journaling:

1. **Be Consistent**: Try to make entries for each music session, even if brief.
2. **Use a Rating System**: To track trends over time, consider using a simple 1-5 scale for mood and engagement.
3. **Include Successes and Challenges**: Note positive responses and difficulties encountered.
4. **Review Regularly**: Set aside time each month to review your journal and look for patterns.

Collaborating with Healthcare Providers on Music Interventions

Healthcare providers can offer valuable insights and support for your music program. Here's how to effectively collaborate with them:

1. **Share Your Observations**: Bring your music therapy journal to appointments to discuss trends and responses.
2. **Ask for Recommendations**: Healthcare providers may suggest specific music or activities based on your loved one's condition.
3. **Discuss Integration with Overall Care Plan**: Explore how music can complement other treatments or therapies.
4. **Address Concerns**: If you notice any negative responses to music, discuss these with the healthcare team.
5. **Consider Professional Music Therapy**: Ask about referrals to certified music therapists for specialized interventions.

Questions to Ask Healthcare Providers:

- How can music support my loved one's specific symptoms or challenges?
- Are there any precautions we should take when using music?
- How often should we reassess our music program?
- Can you recommend resources for expanding our music activities?

Collaborating with Different Healthcare Providers:

Provider	How They Can Help
Neurologist	Insight into how music affects brain function in dementia
Occupational Therapist	Ideas for incorporating music into daily activities
Speech Therapist	Guidance on using music to support communication
Psychiatrist	Advice on using music to manage mood and behavior

Remember, implementing and adjusting a music program is an ongoing process. Be patient with yourself and your loved one as you explore what works best. Celebrate the joyous moments, and don't be discouraged by setbacks – every observation and adjustment brings you closer to an optimal music experience for your loved one.

Your dedication to monitoring and improving your music interventions is genuinely admirable. By carefully observing responses, keeping a detailed journal, and collaborating with healthcare providers, you ensure that your loved one receives the maximum benefit from music in their dementia care. Your efforts can significantly enhance their quality of life and create meaningful moments of connection and joy.

Overcoming Challenges in Music Therapy

As a caregiver or family member of someone with dementia, you may encounter various challenges when implementing music therapy. Understanding how to address these challenges can help you provide your loved one with the most effective and enjoyable musical experiences. Let's explore some common issues and strategies to overcome them.

Dealing with Negative Reactions to Music

While music can be a powerful tool for enhancing mood and cognition, it's essential to be prepared for potential adverse reactions.

Identifying Triggers and Overstimulating Elements

Pay attention to specific aspects of music that may cause distress:

- **Volume**: Too loud or sudden changes in volume
- **Tempo**: Excessively fast or erratic rhythms
- **Lyrics**: Confusing or emotionally charged words
- **Instrumentation**: Harsh or unfamiliar sounds
- **Associations**: Songs linked to unpleasant memories

Techniques for Introducing New or Challenging Music

1. **Gradual Exposure**: Start with short sessions of new music, gradually increasing the duration
2. **Familiar Elements**: Introduce new music that shares characteristics with known favorites
3. **Pairing**: Play new music alongside familiar, enjoyable activities
4. **Choice**: Offer options and respect preferences when introducing new music

When to Stop or Change the Music

Be alert for signs that the music is causing distress:• Increased agitation or anxiety

- Attempts to leave the room or cover ears
- Verbal expressions of discomfort
- Physical signs of stress (e.g., tense muscles, rapid breathing)

If you notice these signs:

1. Immediately stop or change the music
2. Offer reassurance and comfort
3. Switch to a known favorite song or period of quiet
4. Note the incident in your music therapy journal for future reference

Addressing Hearing Impairments

Hearing loss is common in older adults and can impact the effectiveness of music therapy. Here's how to adapt:

Working with Hearing Aids and Music

• Consult with an audiologist to optimize hearing aid settings for music
• Use direct audio input or Bluetooth connectivity when available
• Be mindful of volume levels to prevent discomfort or damage

Alternative Sensory Experiences

When hearing is significantly impaired, consider multi-sensory approaches:

1. **Vibration**:

    • Use bass-heavy speakers or vibrating pillows
    • Encourage feeling the rhythm through touch

2. **Visual Cues**:

    • Incorporate music videos or live performances
    • Use visual rhythm games or apps

3. **Movement**:

    • Encourage dance or rhythmic movement to "feel" the music
    • Use visual cues to guide movement patterns

Communicating with Hearing-Impaired Individuals During Music Activities

• Face the person directly and speak clearly
• Use visual aids like song lyrics or picture cards
• Incorporate hand gestures or simple sign language
• Ensure good lighting for lip-reading if applicable

Managing Overstimulation

People with dementia can be susceptible to sensory input. Here's how to manage overstimulation:

Signs of Sensory Overload

Watch for:
• Increased confusion or disorientation
• Agitation or restlessness
• Covering ears or eyes
• Withdrawal or attempts to leave the environment

Creating a Balanced Sensory Environment

1. **Control the Space**:

    • Minimize background noise
    • Use soft, diffused lighting
    • Remove visual clutter

2. **Timing Matters**:

    • Choose quieter times of day for music activities
    • Avoid introducing music during already stimulating events (e.g., mealtimes)

3. **Personalize the Experience**:

    • Use headphones if environmental sounds are overwhelming
    • Create a dedicated "music corner" with comfortable seating

Techniques for Gradual Exposure to Music

Step	Action	Duration
1	Introduce soft, ambient music	5-10 minutes
2	Gradually increase volume and complexity	Add 5 minutes per session
3	Incorporate simple rhythmic activities	10-15 minutes
4	Slowly extend the session length	Up to 30 minutes
5	Introduce group activities if tolerated	As comfortable

Adapting to Changing Musical Preferences

As dementia progresses, musical preferences may shift. Stay flexible and observant:

Reassessing Music Choices Regularly

• Conduct monthly "music check-ins" to gauge current preferences
• Pay attention to spontaneous reactions to different types of music
• Be open to exploring new genres or styles

Introducing Variety While Maintaining Familiarity

1. **Playlist Rotation**: Create multiple playlists with a mix of familiar and new songs
2. **Theme Days**: Introduce variety through themed music days (e.g., "Classical Mondays," "Jazz Fridays")
3. **Cover Versions**: Play new renditions of familiar songs to bridge the gap between old and new

Respecting Current Preferences vs. Historical Favorites

• Prioritize current positive responses over historical preferences
• Keep a "backup playlist" of all-time favorites for challenging days
• Be willing to let go of music that no longer resonates, even if it was once a favorite

Remember, overcoming challenges in music therapy requires patience, creativity, and a willingness to adapt. Your efforts to tailor the musical experience to your loved one's changing needs are invaluable. By addressing these common issues, you can create a more positive and beneficial music therapy experience, enhancing your loved one's quality of life and strengthening your connection through the power of music.

Music Therapy Resources for Caregivers

As a caregiver for someone with dementia, you've likely experienced the powerful impact music can have on your loved one's mood and cognition. To help you harness the benefits of music therapy, we've compiled a comprehensive list of resources to support your caregiving journey.

Online Music Platforms and Apps

In today's digital age, numerous platforms and apps are designed to make music therapy more accessible and effective for seniors and those with dementia.

Streaming Services with Curated Playlists for Seniors

1. **Spotify**: Offers playlists like "Memories" and "Golden Oldies" specifically curated for seniors.
2. **Apple Music**: Features a "Nostalgia" category with playlists from different decades.
3. **Pandora**: You can create custom stations based on favorite artists or genres from your loved one's youth.

Apps Designed for Dementia Patients and Music Therapy

• **MindMate**: Combines music with brain games and reminiscence activities.
• **Music Memory Box**: You can create personalized playlists linked to photos and memories.
• **SingFit**: Offers lyric prompts and adjustable tempos to encourage singing along.

Free and Low-Cost Music Resources

• **YouTube**: Vast library of free music videos and playlists.
• **Internet Archive**: Offers free access to vintage recordings and radio shows.

• **Local library digital services**: Many libraries offer free access to music streaming platforms.

Support Groups and Forums

Connecting with others who are using music therapy can provide valuable insights and emotional support.

Online Communities for Sharing Music Therapy Experiences

• **Facebook Groups**: Search for "Music Therapy for Dementia" or "Caregivers Using Music."
• **Reddit**: r/musictherapy and r/dementia offer supportive communities.
• **Alzheimer's Association Online Community**: Features a forum for alternative therapies, including music.

Local Support Groups with a Music Focus

1. Contact your local Alzheimer's Association chapter for information on music-focused support groups.

2. Reach out to senior centers or memory care facilities in your area for group activities involving music.

3. Check with local music therapists who may host group sessions or support meetings.

Professional Networks for Caregivers

• **American Music Therapy Association**: Offers resources and networking opportunities for caregivers.
• **Caregiver Action Network**: This network provides a forum for caregivers to connect and share experiences, including those related to music therapy.

Educational Materials and Workshops

Educating yourself about music therapy can enhance your ability to use it effectively in your caregiving routine.

Books and Guides on Music Therapy for Dementia

1. *Connecting Through Music with People with Dementia* by Robin Rio
2. *Music, Memory, and Meaning* by Meredith Hamons, Tara Jenkins, and Cathy Befi-Hensel
3. *Where Memories Go: Why Dementia Changes Everything* by Sally Magnusson

Online Courses and Webinars

• **Coursera**: Offers courses like "Music and the Brain" from the University of Chicago.
• **Udemy**: Features courses on music therapy basics and applications.
• **Music Therapy Ed**: Provides continuing education courses for caregivers and professionals.

Local Workshops and Training Opportunities

1. Check with local colleges or universities with music therapy programs for public workshops.
2. Inquire about caregiver training sessions that include music therapy at senior care facilities.
3. Contact your local Alzheimer's Association for information on upcoming workshops or training events.

Funding and Financial Assistance Options

While music therapy can be a cost-effective intervention, resources are available to help offset any expenses.

Grants and Programs for Music Therapy

• **Music & Memory**: Nonprofit organization that helps bring personalized music to individuals with dementia.
• **NEA Creative Aging Program**: Offers grants for arts programs, including music, for older adults.
• **State Arts Councils**: Many offer grants for therapeutic arts programs.

Insurance Coverage Possibilities

Insurance Type	Potential Coverage
Medicare	May cover music therapy if part of a rehabilitation program
Medicaid	Coverage varies by state; some states include waivers for music therapy in the home and community-based services.
Private Insurance	Some plans cover music therapy under mental health or rehabilitation benefits.

Always check with your specific insurance provider for coverage details.

Crowdfunding and Community Support for Music Programs

1. **GoFundMe**: Create a campaign to fund music therapy sessions or equipment.
2. **DonorsChoose**: For educators or group home staff to request funding for music therapy resources.
3. **Local community foundations** May offer grants or matching funds for innovative care programs.

Remember, implementing music therapy doesn't have to be expensive or complicated. Simple activities like singing together or listening to favorite songs can profoundly impact. Utilizing these resources can enhance your caregiving toolkit and create meaningful musical experiences for your loved one with dementia.

Preparing for End-of-Life Decisions

While difficult to contemplate, preparing for end-of-life decisions is essential to caregiving. Having these conversations and making plans can provide peace of mind and ensure your loved one's wishes are respected.

Steps in Preparing for End-of-Life Decisions:

1. **Start the Conversation**
   - Choose a calm moment to discuss end-of-life wishes with your loved one.
   - Approach the topic with sensitivity and openness.
2. **Understand Your Loved One's Wishes**
   - Discuss preferences for medical interventions, pain management, and place of care.
   - Explore spiritual or cultural considerations.
3. **Document Decisions**
   - Ensure advance directives (living will, healthcare power of attorney) are in place.
   - Consider creating a POLST (Physician Orders for Life-Sustaining Treatment) form.
4. **Communicate with Healthcare Providers**
   - Share documented wishes with all relevant healthcare providers.
   - Ensure copies of advance directives are in medical records.
5. **Plan for Practical Matters**
   - Discuss funeral or memorial preferences.
   - Address financial and legal matters (wills, estate planning).

6. **Prepare Emotionally**
    - Seek support from counselors, support groups, or spiritual advisors.
    - Allow yourself to process emotions as you plan.
7. **Focus on Quality of Life**
    - Discuss what quality of life means to your loved one.
    - Align care decisions with these values.

End-of-Life Consideration	Questions to Discuss	Documentation Needed
Medical Interventions	Preferences for resuscitation, ventilation, feeding tubes	Living Will, POLST Form
Pain Management	Comfort goals, medication preferences	Advance Directive, Pain Management Plan
Place of Care	Preference for home, hospital, or hospice care	Documented in Advance Care Plan
Spiritual/Cultural Needs	Desired rituals, religious support	Noted in Personal Directive

Remember, coping with grief and loss is a profoundly personal journey. There's no right or wrong way to feel; seeking help is okay. By acknowledging your grief, finding meaning in your caregiving role, and preparing for difficult decisions, you're honoring both yourself and your loved one.

These conversations and preparations, while challenging, can bring a sense of peace and allow you to focus on creating meaningful moments with your loved one. Don't hesitate to lean on your support network, seek professional help if needed, and be gentle with yourself throughout this process. Your role as a caregiver is invaluable, and taking care of your emotional well-being is essential to providing compassionate care.

.

When to Consider Hospice

Hospice care is a compassionate approach to end-of-life care that focuses on comfort, quality of life, and dignity. It's important to understand that choosing hospice doesn't mean giving up – it means shifting the focus from curative treatment to comfort care.

Critical aspects of hospice care include:

1. Pain management and symptom control
2. Emotional and spiritual support for the patient and family
3. Assistance with personal care and daily living activities
4. Respite care for family caregivers
5. Bereavement support for loved ones

Hospice care is typically provided by a team of professionals, including:

- Doctors
- Nurses
- Social workers
- Chaplains or spiritual advisors
- Trained volunteers

Hospice Service	Description
Medical Care	Pain management, symptom control, and medication management.
Personal Care	Assistance with bathing, dressing, and other daily activities.
Emotional Support	Counseling for patient and family, addressing fears and concerns.
Spiritual Care	Support for spiritual needs and end-of-life rituals.
Practical Support	Help with household tasks, errands, and respite care.

The importance of timely hospice involvement

Deciding when to involve hospice care can be emotionally challenging, but **early involvement often leads to better outcomes** for both the person with dementia and their caregivers. Here's why timely hospice care is crucial:

1. **Improved quality of life**: Hospice teams are experts in managing pain and other symptoms, helping your loved one feel more comfortable.
2. **Reduced hospitalizations**: Proper symptom management often reduces the need for emergency room visits or hospital stays.
3. **Emotional and spiritual support**: Hospice offers counseling and support services that benefit you and your loved one.
4. **Time to say goodbye**: Earlier involvement gives family members more time to spend with their loved one and address unfinished business.
5. **Caregiver support**: Hospice provides education, resources, and respite care to help you navigate this challenging time.

Remember, choosing hospice doesn't mean death is imminent. Many patients receive hospice care for months, allowing them to make the most of their remaining time with improved comfort and quality of life.

Benefits of Early Hospice Involvement	Impact on Patient and Family
Better symptom management	Increased comfort and reduced suffering
Comprehensive support	Improved overall quality of life for the patient and caregivers
Avoid crises	Less stress and anxiety for family members
Time for meaningful moments	Opportunity to create lasting memories and say goodbyes

By understanding dementia, hospice care, and the benefits of timely involvement, you're better equipped to make informed decisions about your loved one's care. Remember, you're not alone in this journey – hospice teams are there to support both you and your loved one every step of the way.

Signs It May Be Time for Hospice Care

As a caregiver or family member of someone with dementia, recognizing when it's time to consider hospice care can be challenging. This decision is deeply personal and often emotional. However, certain signs can help guide you in making this vital choice. Let's explore these indicators in detail.

Physical indicators

Physical changes are often the most noticeable signs that your loved one's condition is progressing. **Look for these physical indicators**:

1. **Significant weight loss**: A 10% or more decrease in body weight in six months.
2. **Frequent infections**: Pneumonia or urinary tract infections that are becoming harder to treat.
3. **Difficulty swallowing**: This can lead to choking, coughing during meals, or refusal to eat.
4. **Increased pain**: Despite efforts to manage it with medication.
5. **Skin breakdown**: Pressure sores or other skin issues that aren't healing.
6. **Changes in breathing**: Shortness of breath, labored breathing, or long pauses between breaths.
7. **Decreased mobility**: Becoming bed-bound or unable to sit up without support.

Physical Indicator	What to Look For
Weight Loss	Loose clothing, visible bone structure, sunken cheeks
Swallowing Difficulties	Coughing during meals, holding food in the mouth, refusing to eat
Skin Issues	Redness, open sores, slow healing of wounds
Mobility Changes	Inability to walk independently, frequent falls, reluctance to move

Cognitive and behavioral changes

As dementia progresses, you may notice significant changes in your loved one's cognitive abilities and behavior. **Fundamental changes to watch for include**:

- Increased confusion and disorientation
- Difficulty recognizing family members
- Loss of ability to communicate verbally
- Agitation, aggression, or combative behavior
- Withdrawal from social interactions
- Changes in sleep patterns (sleeping more during the day, restless at night)
- Hallucinations or delusions

Remember, these changes can be distressing for you and your loved one. Hospice care can help you manage these symptoms and improve your quality of life.

Frequent hospitalizations or ER visits

If you find yourself taking your loved one to the emergency room or hospital more often, it might be time to consider hospice care. **Signs to consider include**:

1. Multiple hospitalizations within the past six months
2. Recurring infections or illnesses
3. Increasing difficulty managing symptoms at home
4. Longer recovery times after each hospital stay

Frequency of Medical Visits	Consideration
1-2 ER visits in 6 months	Monitor closely and consult with a doctor.
3+ ER visits in 6 months	This is a strong indication for a hospice evaluation.
Any hospital stay longer than one week	Consider hospice discussion.

Decline in daily functioning

A significant decline in your loved one's ability to perform daily tasks independently is a strong indicator that hospice care may be beneficial. **Watch for**:

- Inability to dress, bathe, or groom without assistance
- Incontinence or loss of bladder and bowel control
- Difficulty moving from bed to chair without help
- Inability to prepare or eat meals independently
- Decreased interest in previously enjoyed activities

These changes often mean that your loved one requires more intensive care, which hospice can provide while ensuring comfort and dignity.

In conclusion, deciding when to consider hospice care is complex and personal. By being aware of these signs – physical changes, cognitive decline, frequent hospitalizations, and decreased daily functioning – you can make a more informed choice about when to seek additional support. Remember, hospice care is not about giving up hope; it's about ensuring the best possible quality of life for your loved one and support for you as a caregiver.

The Benefits of Hospice Care for Dementia Patients

When considering hospice care for your loved one with dementia, it's essential to understand the numerous benefits this specialized care can provide. Hospice focuses on comfort and quality of life, offering a holistic approach to supporting the patient and their family. Let's explore these benefits in detail.

Pain management and symptom control

One of the primary goals of hospice care is to ensure that your loved one is as comfortable as possible. **Effective pain management and symptom control can significantly improve their quality of life.**

Critical aspects of pain and symptom management in hospice care include:

1. **Personalized pain assessment**: Hospice professionals are trained to recognize pain in patients who cannot communicate verbally.
2. **Tailored medication plans**: Medications are carefully selected and adjusted to provide maximum comfort with minimal side effects.
3. **Non-pharmacological interventions** may include massage, music therapy, or aromatherapy to complement medication.
4. **Regular monitoring**: The hospice team assesses the patient's comfort level and adjusts care as needed.
5. **Management of other symptoms**: This includes addressing issues like shortness of breath, nausea, anxiety, and sleep disturbances.

Common Dementia Symptoms	Hospice Management Approach
Pain	Tailored pain medication, positioning, gentle massage
Agitation	Calming techniques, environmental adjustments, medication if necessary
Difficulty swallowing	Dietary modifications, proper positioning, oral care
Skin issues	Regular repositioning, specialized mattresses, wound care

Emotional and spiritual support

Hospice care recognizes that emotional and spiritual well-being is as important as physical comfort. **This holistic approach can provide immense comfort to the patient and their family.**

Emotional and spiritual support in hospice care includes:

- Counseling services for the patient and family members
- Support from social workers to address practical and emotional concerns
- Chaplain services for spiritual support, regardless of religious affiliation
- Assistance with life review and legacy projects
- Grief counseling for family members, both before and after their loved one's passing

Remember, this support is tailored to your family's needs and beliefs. The hospice team is there to provide comfort and guidance, not to impose any particular spiritual or religious views.

Respite care for family caregivers

Caring for a loved one with dementia can be physically and emotionally exhausting. **Hospice care recognizes the vital role of family caregivers and offers respite services to prevent burnout.**

Respite care benefits include:

1. Short-term relief from caregiving duties
2. Opportunity for self-care and rest
3. Time to attend to personal matters or other family responsibilities
4. Professional care for your loved one, ensuring their needs are met
5. Reduced stress and improved overall well-being for the caregiver

Improved quality of life

The ultimate goal of hospice care is to improve the patient's and their family's overall quality of life. **This is achieved through expert care, support, and a focus on comfort rather than curative treatments.**

Ways hospice care can improve quality of life:

- Allowing the patient to remain in familiar surroundings, often at home
- Providing equipment and supplies necessary for comfort and care
- Offering 24/7 support and guidance for family caregivers
- Facilitating meaningful interactions and moments between the patient and their loved ones
- Ensuring dignity and respect in all aspects of care

Addressing not just physical needs but also emotional, social, and spiritual needs Quality of Life Aspect	Hospice Care Impact
Comfort	Reduced pain and distressing symptoms.
Dignity	Personalized care respecting individual preferences.
Family connection	Support for meaningful interactions and memory-making.
Peace of mind	24/7 professional support and guidance.

In conclusion, hospice care offers numerous benefits for dementia patients and their families. By focusing on comprehensive symptom management, providing emotional and spiritual support, offering respite care, and striving to improve overall quality of life, hospice care can make a significant difference in your loved one's final months or years.

Remember, choosing hospice care doesn't mean giving up hope. Instead, it means shifting the focus to ensuring the best possible quality of life and comfort for your loved one. It's about making the most of your time together, creating meaningful moments, and finding peace in knowing your loved one receives expert, compassionate care.

Common Misconceptions About Hospice Care

When considering hospice care for a loved one with dementia, you may encounter several misconceptions that can cause hesitation or concern. Understanding the realities of hospice care is essential to making an informed decision. Let's address the most common misconceptions and clarify what hospice care entails.

Hospice is not giving up.

One of the most pervasive misconceptions about hospice care is that it means "giving up" on your loved one. **This couldn't be further from the truth.**

Here's why hospice is not giving up:

1. **Shift in focus**: Hospice represents a change in care goals, not an abandonment of care. The focus shifts from curative treatments to comfort and quality of life.
2. **Active care**: Hospice provides expert care to manage symptoms and improve comfort.
3. **A holistic approach** addresses not just physical needs but also emotional, social, and spiritual aspects of well-being.
4. **Empowerment**: Hospice empowers patients and families to make choices about their care and how they want to spend their remaining time.
5. **Celebration of life**: Many hospice programs encourage life reviews and legacy projects, which celebrate the person's life and accomplishments.

Misconception	Reality
Hospice means no more treatment.	Hospice provides active treatment for symptoms and comfort.
Choosing hospice means giving up hope.	Hospice shifts hope to quality of life and meaningful moments.
Hospice is only for the last few days of life.	Hospice can provide care for months, enhancing life quality.

Hospice doesn't mean imminent death.

Another common misconception is that hospice care is only for the last few days or weeks of life. **Hospice care can be beneficial for months and sometimes even longer.**

Key points to understand:

- Hospice eligibility typically requires a prognosis of six months or less, but this is not a strict limit.
- Many patients receive hospice care for several months, with some even "graduating" from hospice if their condition stabilizes.
- Earlier involvement of hospice often leads to a better quality of life and can sometimes even extend life by reducing stress on the body.
- Hospice care can be discontinued if the patient's condition improves or if they decide to pursue curative treatments again.

Time in Hospice	Potential Benefits
Days to weeks	Immediate comfort care and family support in crisis
Weeks to months	Sustained symptom management, quality time with family
Months or longer	Long-term comfort, potential for stabilization or improvement

Hospice care can be provided at home.

Many people believe that choosing hospice care means their loved one must move to a facility. **Hospice care is often provided right in the comfort of the patient's home.**

Understanding home hospice care:

1. **Flexibility**: Hospice care can be provided wherever the patient calls home – private residences, assisted living facilities, or nursing homes.
2. **Customized care**: The hospice team works with you to create a care plan that fits your home environment and family dynamics.
3. **Equipment and supplies**: Necessary medical equipment (like hospital beds or oxygen) is provided and set up in the home.

4. **24/7 support**: While the hospice team isn't present 24/7, they're always available by phone for guidance and can visit as needed.
5. **Family involvement**: Home hospice allows family members to be intimately involved in care, with guidance from the hospice team.
6. **Familiar surroundings**: Patients often find comfort surrounded by familiar sights, sounds, and loved ones.

Aspect of Care	In-Home Hospice Provision
Medical care	Regular visits from nurses and doctors
Personal care	Assistance with bathing and dressing by hospice aides
Emotional support	Visits from social workers and counselors
Spiritual care	Chaplain visits if desired

It's important to note that while home hospice is common, inpatient hospice facilities are available for those who need or prefer that option. Some patients may transition between home and inpatient care as their needs change.

In conclusion, understanding these common misconceptions about hospice care can help you make a more informed decision for your loved one with dementia. Hospice is not about giving up or waiting for death; it's about living life as fully and comfortably as possible in whatever time remains. It offers expert care that can often be provided at home, surrounding your loved one with familiar comforts and loving family members.

Remember, choosing hospice care is a profoundly personal decision. It's okay to have questions and concerns. Don't hesitate to contact hospice providers in your area to learn more about their services and how they might benefit your loved one and your family. Your choice to consider hospice care demonstrates your commitment to ensuring the best possible quality of life for your loved one, which is an act of profound love and care.

How to Initiate the Hospice Conversation

Initiating a conversation about hospice care can be challenging and emotionally charged. However, having these discussions early can lead to better care decisions and more time to prepare. Here's how to approach this sensitive topic with compassion and clarity.

Talking with your loved one

When possible, it's essential to involve your loved one with dementia in the decision-making process. While their ability to participate may vary, including them shows respect for their wishes and autonomy.

Tips for talking with your loved one:

1. **Choose the right time and place**: Find a quiet, comfortable setting where your loved one is most alert and receptive.
2. **Be direct but gentle**: Use clear, simple language. Avoid euphemisms that might confuse them.
3. **Listen actively**: Pay attention to their verbal and non-verbal responses.
4. **Respect their feelings**: Acknowledge any fears or concerns they express.
5. **Focus on the benefits**: Explain how hospice can help manage their symptoms and improve comfort.
6. **Be patient.** This may need to be an ongoing conversation. Don't rush to decide everything in one sitting.

Use visual aids: If appropriate, consider using brochures or videos to help explain hospice care. What to Say	**What to Avoid**
"I want to talk about how we can keep you comfortable."	"We need to discuss end-of-life care."
"Hospice can help us manage your pain better."	"There's nothing more we can do for you."
"What's most important to you right now?"	"You should consider hospice care."

Discussing with family members

Bringing up hospice care with other family members can sometimes be as challenging as discussing it with your loved one. Family dynamics, differing opinions, and emotional responses can complicate these conversations.

Strategies for family discussions:

- **Plan**: Consider who should be part of the conversation and how to involve distant family members.
- **Choose a spokesperson**: Designate one person to lead the conversation if helpful.
- **Share information**: Before the discussion, provide educational materials about hospice care to all family members.
- **Be inclusive**: Ensure everyone has a chance to express their thoughts and feelings.
- **Focus on your loved one's wishes**: If known, center the discussion on what your loved one with dementia would want.
- **Address concerns**: Be open to questions and address fears or misconceptions about hospice care.

Seek professional help: Consider involving a social worker or counselor to facilitate the conversation if family conflicts arise. **Common Family Concerns**	**Possible Responses**
"Isn't this giving up?"	"Hospice focuses on quality of life and comfort, not giving up."
"It's too soon to consider hospice."	"Earlier hospice involvement often leads to better care and support."
"We can't afford it."	"Medicare, Medicaid, and most private insurances usually cover hospice."

Consulting with healthcare providers

Healthcare providers play a crucial role in the decision to pursue hospice care. They can provide valuable insights into your loved one's condition and prognosis and help you understand if hospice is appropriate.

Steps for consulting healthcare providers:

1. **Schedule a dedicated appointment**: Request a meeting to discuss your loved one's care options, including hospice.
2. **Prepare questions**: Write down your questions and concerns beforehand. Some key questions might include:
   - Is my loved one eligible for hospice care?
   - How might hospice benefit them at this stage?
   - What changes in their condition should we be watching for?
3. **Bring support**: Consider having another family member present to help remember information.
4. **Take notes**: Write down important points or ask if you can record the conversation for future reference.

5. **Discuss prognosis**: While difficult, understanding the expected progression of your loved one's condition can help you make decisions.
6. **Ask about referrals**: If hospice seems appropriate, ask for referrals to reputable hospice providers in your area.
7. **Follow-up**: Don't hesitate to contact the healthcare provider with any additional questions after the meeting.

Healthcare Provider	Role in Hospice Discussion
Primary Care Physician	Overall health assessment and long-term care planning.
Neurologist	Dementia progression and symptom management.
Geriatrician	Specialized care needs for older adults.
Palliative Care Specialist	Expert in comfort care and quality of life issues.

Remember, initiating the hospice conversation is an act of love and care. It shows that you're thinking proactively about ensuring the best possible quality of life for your loved one. While these discussions can be difficult, they often bring a sense of relief and clarity once they're underway.

It's normal to feel a range of emotions during this process. Don't hesitate to seek support for yourself, whether from friends, support groups, or professional counselors. Taking care of your emotional well-being is crucial as you navigate this challenging journey.

Ultimately, the goal is to make informed decisions that honor your loved one's wishes and provide them with the most appropriate and compassionate care possible. By approaching these conversations with openness, empathy, and a focus on your loved one's well-being, you can navigate this critical decision-making process with greater confidence and peace of mind.

The Hospice Evaluation Process

Understanding the hospice evaluation process can help alleviate some of the anxiety and uncertainty you may feel when considering this option for your loved one with dementia. This process ensures that hospice care is appropriate and tailored to your loved one's specific needs. Let's explore each step in detail.

Eligibility criteria for dementia patients

Specific criteria apply to people with dementia who are eligible for hospice care. **These criteria are guidelines, and each case is evaluated individually**.

Key eligibility factors for dementia patients include:

1. **Disease progression**: The person should be in the late stages of dementia, typically stage 7, on the Functional Assessment Staging Test (FAST).
2. **Functional decline**: Inability to perform daily activities without substantial assistance.
3. **Medical complications**: Presence of conditions such as aspiration pneumonia, upper urinary tract infections, sepsis, or multiple stage 3-4 pressure ulcers.
4. **Nutritional decline**: Difficulty eating and swallowing, leading to weight loss.
5. **Verbal communication**: Limited to fewer than six intelligible daily words.
6. **Mobility**: Unable to walk without assistance and eventually becoming bed-bound.

Eligibility Factor	Description
FAST Stage 7	Very severe cognitive decline, minimal verbal communication
ADL Dependence	Requires help with most or all activities of daily living
Medical Complications	Recurrent infections, difficulty swallowing, pressure sores
Nutritional Decline	Significant weight loss, difficulty eating independently

Remember, meeting these criteria doesn't automatically mean hospice is the right choice, nor does failing to meet all requirements necessarily disqualify someone. The decision involves a comprehensive evaluation by healthcare professionals and discussions with the family.

What to expect during the evaluation

The hospice evaluation is a thorough process designed to assess your loved one's needs and determine whether hospice care is appropriate. **It is typically provided at no cost and does not obligate you to choose hospice care**.

The evaluation process usually includes:

- **Initial consultation**: A hospice representative will meet with you and your loved one to explain services and answer questions.
- **Medical review**: The hospice team will review your loved one's medical history and condition.
- **Physical assessment**: A nurse will conduct a physical examination to evaluate symptoms and care needs.
- **Psychosocial assessment**: A social worker may assess emotional needs and family dynamics.
- **Home safety evaluation**: If care will be provided at home, the team will assess the environment for safety and equipment needs.
- **Discussion of goals**: The team will discuss your loved one's care goals and preferences with you.

Evaluation Step	Conducted By
Initial Consultation	Hospice Representative
Medical Review	Hospice Physician
Physical Assessment	Hospice Nurse
Psychosocial Assessment	Social Worker

Creating a care plan

If your loved one is found eligible for hospice and you decide to proceed, the next step is creating a personalized care plan. This plan is a **collaborative effort** between the hospice team, your loved one (if able to participate), and your family.

The care plan typically includes:

1. **Symptom management strategies**: Plans for managing pain, anxiety, breathing difficulties, and other symptoms.
2. **Medication regimen**: A review and adjustment of current medications, focusing on comfort and symptom control.
3. **Personal care routines**: Plans for bathing, feeding, and other daily care needs.
4. **Emotional and spiritual support**: Arrange counseling, chaplain visits, or other support services.
5. **Family education**: Training for family caregivers on providing care and recognizing important signs or symptoms.
6. **Emergency procedures**: Clear instructions on what to do in case of emergencies or sudden changes in condition.
7. **Respite care arrangements**: Plans for providing breaks to family caregivers.

Care Plan Component	Purpose
Symptom Management	Ensure comfort and quality of life.
Medication Management	Optimize effectiveness and minimize side effects.
Personal Care	Maintain dignity and prevent complications.
Emotional Support	Address the psychological needs of the patient and family.

It's important to understand that the care plan is a **dynamic document**. It will be regularly reviewed and adjusted as your loved one's needs change. You and your family will be integral parts of this ongoing process.

Remember, the hospice evaluation and care planning process ensures your loved one receives the most appropriate and compassionate care possible. It's an opportunity to ask questions, express concerns, and actively participate in shaping your loved one's care.

Don't hesitate to ask for clarification if anything is unclear during this process. The hospice team supports you and your loved one every step of the way. They aim to honor your loved one's wishes, provide expert care, and help your entire family through this challenging time.

By understanding and actively participating in the evaluation and care planning process, you're taking an essential step in ensuring the best possible care and quality of life for your loved one with dementia. While sometimes emotional, this process can also bring relief and clarity as you navigate this difficult journey.

Preparing for Hospice Care

Once you've decided to pursue hospice care for your loved one with dementia, there are several important steps to take to ensure a smooth transition. This preparation phase is crucial for creating a supportive environment and understanding what to expect. Let's explore these steps in detail.

Choosing a Hospice Provider

Selecting the right hospice provider is a critical decision that can significantly impact the quality of care your loved one receives. **Take your time with this process, and don't hesitate to ask questions.**

Consider the following when choosing a hospice provider:

1. **Certification and accreditation**: Ensure the provider is Medicare-certified and, ideally, accredited by a national organization.
2. **Range of services**: Look for providers offering comprehensive medical, emotional, and spiritual support.
3. **Availability**: Choose a provider that offers 24/7 emergency on-call services.

4. **Experience with dementia**: Ask about their specific experience in caring for patients with dementia.
5. **Staff qualifications**: Inquire about the training and qualifications of their care team members.
6. **Respite care options**: Check if they offer respite care to give family caregivers breaks.
7. **Bereavement support**: Look for providers that offer grief counseling and support after your loved one's passing.

Question to Ask	Why It's Important
How quickly can you start services?	Ensures timely care initiation
What is your staff-to-patient ratio?	Indicates the level of individual attention
How do you manage pain in dementia patients?	Reveals expertise in dementia-specific care
What support do you offer family caregivers?	Indicates the level of family involvement and support

Setting up the care environment

Creating a safe, comfortable environment is essential for hospice care, especially if your loved one will be cared for at home. **The goal is to promote comfort, safety, and ease of care.**

Critical considerations for setting up the care environment:

- **Bedroom setup**: Ensure the bed is accessible from both sides. If recommended by the hospice team, consider a hospital bed.
- **Bathroom modifications**: Install grab bars, a raised toilet seat, and non-slip mats if needed.
- **Clear pathways**: Remove clutter and ensure clear paths for easy movement, primarily if a wheelchair or walker is used.
- **Lighting**: Provide adequate lighting to prevent falls and aid in care tasks.

- **Comfortable seating**: Have a comfortable chair for your loved one and seating for visitors.
- **Temperature control**: Ensure the room can be kept at a comfortable temperature.
- **Meaningful objects**: Include photos, favorite blankets, or other cherished items to create a comforting atmosphere.

Item	Purpose
Hospital bed	Allows for positioning adjustments, easier care
Bedside commode	Reduces the need for bathroom trips
Over-bed table	Provides surface for meals, activities
Night light	Improves safety during nighttime care

Understanding your role as a caregiver

As a family caregiver, your role will evolve with the introduction of hospice care. **While the hospice team will provide expert care, your involvement remains crucial.**

Your role as a caregiver may include:

1. **Being an advocate**: You know your loved one best. Share insights about their preferences, behaviors, and needs with the hospice team.
2. **Providing comfort**: Your presence and touch can be incredibly comforting. Spend time with your loved one, hold their hand, or sit with them.
3. **Assisting with personal care**: The hospice team will guide you in helping with feeding, bathing, or repositioning.
4. **Medication management**: While the hospice team will manage medications, you may be involved in administering them.
5. **Emotional support**: Provide reassurance and emotional support to your loved one.
6. **Communication liaison**: Keep other family members informed about your loved one's condition and care.

7. **Self-care**: Remember to take care of yourself too. Accept help and take breaks when needed.

Caregiver Task	Hospice Team Support
Personal care assistance	Training on safe techniques, along with regular help from hospice aides
Medication administration	Clear instructions, regular check-ins, 24/7 phone support
Emotional support	Counseling services, tips for communication
Recognizing changes in condition	Education on what to watch for, when to call for help

Remember, the hospice team supports you and your loved one. **Don't hesitate to ask for help or clarification when you need it.** They can provide training, answer questions, and support you as you navigate this new role.

Preparing for hospice care can feel overwhelming, but taking these steps can help create a smoother transition. By choosing the right provider, setting up a comfortable environment, and understanding your role, you're laying the groundwork for compassionate, quality care for your loved one.

This preparation phase is also a time for emotional readiness. It's normal to feel a mix of emotions – relief, sadness, anxiety, or even guilt. Remember that choosing hospice care is an act of love, focusing on comfort and quality of life for your loved one. Don't hesitate to lean on the hospice team, friends, or support groups for emotional support.

By taking these steps to prepare, you're ensuring that your loved one will receive the best possible care in their final stage of life while also setting yourself up to be an informed and supported caregiver. Your dedication to this process is a testament to your love and commitment to your family member's well-being.

Navigating the Emotional Journey

The decision to pursue hospice care for a loved one with dementia marks the beginning of a profound emotional journey. This period can be filled with complex feelings and challenges. Understanding these emotions and finding coping methods is crucial for you and your loved one. Let's explore this journey and discuss strategies for navigating it with resilience and grace.

Coping with grief and anticipatory loss

Grief is a natural response to loss, and it often begins well before the actual passing of a loved one. This is known as anticipatory grief. **Recognizing and acknowledging these feelings is an essential step in coping with them.**

Common experiences of anticipatory grief include:

- Sadness and tearfulness
- Anxiety about the future
- Anger or frustration
- Guilt over past events or current feelings
- A sense of helplessness
- Difficulty concentrating
- Physical symptoms like fatigue or changes in appetite

Strategies for coping with anticipatory grief:

1. **Acknowledge your feelings**: Allow yourself to feel whatever emotions arise without judgment.
2. **Share your feelings**: Talk to trusted friends, family members, or a professional counselor.
3. **Practice self-compassion**: Be kind to yourself. Grief is a normal and valid response to your situation.
4. **Stay connected**: Maintain relationships with friends and family. Don't isolate yourself.
5. **Take care of your physical health**: Eat well, exercise, and get enough sleep.
6. **Find healthy outlets**: Engage in activities that help you process your emotions, such as journaling, art, or music.

7. **Stay present**: While worrying about the future is natural, focus on the present moment and your time with your loved one.

Grief Response	Coping Strategy
Overwhelming sadness	Allow yourself to cry; talk to a supportive friend.
Anxiety about the future	Practice mindfulness; focus on one day at a time.
Guilt over negative feelings	Practice self-compassion; join a support group.
Physical exhaustion	Prioritize self-care; ask for help with tasks.

Finding support for caregivers

Caring for a loved one with dementia in hospice care can be emotionally and physically demanding. **Seeking support is not a sign of weakness but a necessary step in maintaining your well-being.**

Options for caregiver support include:

- **Support groups**: Join groups specifically for dementia caregivers or hospice families. These can be in-person or online.
- **Professional counseling**: Consider individual therapy to process emotions and develop coping strategies.
- **Respite care**: Take your hospice provider's respite services for necessary breaks.
- **Family and friends**: Don't hesitate to ask for and accept help from your support network.
- **Educational resources**: Attend workshops or webinars about caregiving and end-of-life care to feel more prepared.
- **Spiritual or religious support**: If applicable, seek guidance from spiritual leaders or faith communities.
- **Self-care activities**: Engage in activities that recharge you, even for short periods.

Type of Support	Benefits
Caregiver support groups	Shared experiences, practical tips, emotional validation.
Professional counseling	Personalized coping strategies and safe space to process emotions.
Respite care	Time for self-care and reduced burnout risk.
Educational resources	Increased confidence in caregiving, better preparedness.

Celebrating life and creating meaningful moments

While this time is undoubtedly challenging, it also presents opportunities to celebrate your loved one's life and create lasting memories. **Focusing on positive experiences can provide comfort and meaning during this challenging journey.**

Ideas for creating meaningful moments:

1. **Life review**: Remember happy memories, perhaps creating a scrapbook or memory box together.
2. **Music therapy**: Play your loved one's favorite songs or hymns. Music can often evoke positive responses, even in late-stage dementia.
3. **Sensory experiences**: Engage the senses with familiar scents, textures, or flavors that bring comfort.
4. **Nature connection**: If possible, spend time outdoors or bring nature inside with flowers or plants.
5. **Gentle touch**: Hold hands, give a soft massage, or sit close to provide comfort through touch.
6. **Family gatherings**: Organize small, quiet gatherings of close family and friends to share stories and love.
7. **Legacy projects**: Create something together that can be shared with future generations, like a recipe book or family tree.
8. **Spiritual practices**: If prayer, meditation, or other spiritual practices are essential to your loved one, engage in them.

Meaningful Activity	Potential Benefits
Looking at old photos	Stimulates memories and encourages storytelling.
Listening to favorite music	It evokes emotions and may improve mood.
Gentle hand massage	It provides comfort and promotes relaxation.
Reading aloud familiar stories	Offers comfort and maintains connection.

Remember, the goal is not to create grand gestures but to find moments of connection, comfort, and joy, however small they seem.

Navigating the emotional journey of hospice care for a loved one with dementia is undoubtedly challenging. It's a path filled with complex emotions, difficult decisions, and profound moments of love and connection. You can find strength and moments of peace by acknowledging your feelings, seeking support, and focusing on creating meaningful experiences.

It's important to remember that there's no "right" way to feel or grieve. Your journey is unique, and having good and bad days is okay. Be patient and compassionate with yourself as you navigate this path.

Lastly, don't forget that the hospice team supports you and your loved one. They can provide resources, counseling, and guidance to help you through this emotional journey. You're not alone in this process; reaching out for help when needed is a sign of strength and love for yourself and your loved one.

Legal and Financial Considerations

When caring for a loved one with dementia who is entering hospice care, it's important to consider legal and financial matters. These can be challenging topics, but planning can bring peace of mind and help avoid problems later. Let's look at some key things to consider.

Advance Directives and Power of Attorney

Advance directives say what kind of medical care your loved one wants if they can't speak for themselves. There are two main types:

1. Living Will: This document states what medical treatments your loved one wants or doesn't want at the end of life.
2. Healthcare Power of Attorney: This names someone to make medical decisions if your loved one can't.

Power of attorney is also crucial for money matters. It lets someone manage your loved one's finances if they can't do it themselves.

Why these papers matter:

- They make sure your loved one's wishes are followed
- They can prevent family arguments about care decisions
- They make it easier to handle bills and other money matters

Setting these up early is best while your loved one can still make decisions. If you haven't done this yet, talk to a lawyer who knows about elder law as soon as possible.

Document	What It Does
Living Will	States end-of-life care wishes
Healthcare Power of Attorney	Names someone to make medical decisions
Financial Power of Attorney	Names someone to handle money matters

Understanding Hospice Coverage and Costs

The good news is that Medicare, Medicaid, and most private insurance plans usually cover hospice care. This coverage includes:

- Doctor and nursing services
- Medical equipment and supplies
- Medications for symptom control and pain relief
- Short-term inpatient care, if needed
- Grief counseling for the patient and family

What's not covered:

- Room and board if the patient is at home or in a nursing facility
- Treatments aimed at curing the illness (instead of comfort care); such treatments can invalidate hospice services.

It's good to check with your hospice provider and insurance company to understand what's covered and what you might need to pay for.

Usually Covered	Usually Not Covered
Hospice team visits	Curative treatments (which can invalidate hospice services)
Medical equipment	Room and board at home
Medications for comfort	Care from providers outside the hospice

Additional Resources and Support Programs

Besides insurance, other programs might help with costs or provide extra support:

1. Veterans Benefits: If your loved one served in the military, they might qualify for special hospice benefits through the VA.
2. Social Security: Your loved one might be eligible for disability benefits if they're under 65.
3. Local Senior Services: Many communities have programs that offer seniors meals, transportation, or other help.
4. Alzheimer's Association: They offer support groups and education and can help you find local resources.
5. Area Agency on Aging: This government program can connect you with services in your area.

Don't be afraid to ask for help. Social workers at the hospice or your local senior center can often recommend programs that might help.

Resource	What It Offers
Veterans Benefits	Special hospice care for veterans
Social Security	Possible disability benefits
Alzheimer's Association	Support groups and education

Remember, dealing with legal and money matters can feel overwhelming, but it's integral to caring for your loved one. Don't hesitate to ask for help from professionals like lawyers, financial advisors, or social workers. They can guide you through these complex issues and help you make the best decisions for your family.

Conclusion

As we reach the end of our journey through "Music Therapy for Dementia: A Dementia Care Essentials Guide," I hope you've discovered the transformative power of music in dementia care. Music has the unique ability to touch hearts, awaken memories, and bring moments of joy even in the most challenging times.

Remember, you don't need to be a professional musician or therapist to bring music's benefits into your loved one's life. Whether you're singing a familiar tune, playing a favorite record, or simply tapping out a rhythm together, every musical moment you create is a gift of connection and comfort.

As you move forward in your caregiving journey, I encourage you to embrace music as a tool for communication, emotional expression, and memory stimulation. Be patient with yourself and your loved one as you explore what works best for you both. Celebrate the small victories – a smile, a tapped foot, or a moment of recognition – as these are precious triumphs in the world of dementia care.

Don't be afraid to seek support when you need it. Whether you consult with a professional music therapist, join a support group, or simply share your experiences with friends and family, remember that you're not alone in this journey.

Caring for someone with dementia is undoubtedly challenging, but it can also be a profoundly rewarding experience. By incorporating music into your care routine, you're not just managing symptoms – you're creating opportunities for meaningful connection, emotional expression, and moments of pure joy.

As you close this book, I hope you feel empowered to bring the healing power of music into your caregiving journey. Your dedication to enhancing your loved one's quality of life through music is truly admirable. Remember, every note you share is a testament to your love and commitment.

Thank you for allowing me to be a part of your caregiving journey. May the music you share with your loved one bring comfort, joy, and beautiful moments of connection in the days ahead.

Resources

Associations

Alzheimer's Association at https://www.alz.org/

Dementia Society of America at http://www.dementiasociety.org

National Institute on Aging at https://www.nia.nih.gov/

National Alliance for Caregiving at http://www.caregiving.org

Family Caregiver Alliance at http://www.caregiver.org

American Sleep Apnea Association at https://www.sleepapnea.org/

Author Bio

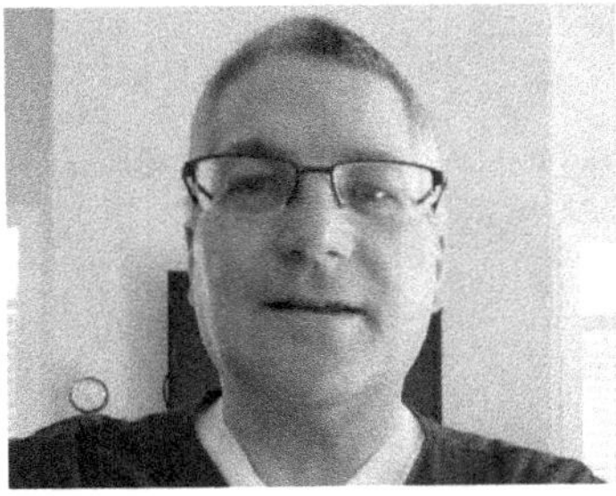

Peter Abraham, BSN, RN is an experienced nurse dedicated to supporting nurses, caregivers, families, and patients in their learning, growth, and well-being journey. Peter's nursing path encompasses practical experience as a cardiac telemetry nurse in a bustling cardiology unit at a Magnet-awarded teaching hospital. Additionally, Peter has fulfilled the role of a second-shift RN supervisor, overseeing an entire building in an SNF/LTC (Skilled Nursing Facility/Long-Term Care) setting with 151 residents. Remarkably, during the initial wave of COVID-19, the facility achieved an impressive close-to-100% recovery rate before operation warp speed was complete.

Furthermore, Peter's nursing career extends to rural home hospice care. As a visiting hospice registered nurse case manager, he offers compassionate care to patients in various settings, including private homes, personal care homes, assisted living facilities, skilled nursing facilities, and hospitals.

Moreover, Peter's desire to help others extends beyond his physical presence. At CompassionCrossing.Info, he writes articles to empower caregivers, family members, and fellow nurses in end-of-life care. Peter's drive to help others, which flows from his love of Christ Jesus, is a source of support and encouragement for all he reaches.

Other books by Peter Abraham include the following:

Empowering Excellence in Hospice: A Nurse's Toolkit for Best Practices series:

Compliance-based, Eligibility Driven Hospice Documentation: Tips for Hospice Nurses
Whispers of Time: Understanding the End-of-Life Timeline
Terminal Clarity: Hospice Eligibility Guide for Nurses

Compassionate Caregiving series:

Daily Hospice Care Planner: Organize, Communicate, and Provide Consistent Care
Dignity in Dying: A Thoughtful Approach to Voluntary Stopping Eating and Drinking
Palliative Sedation: A Compassionate Approach
Hospice Medication Handbook: A Caregiver's Guide to Comfort Medications

Dementia Caregivers Essentials series:

CPAP and Oxygen for Dementia
Diabetes Care for Dementia
Hallucination Management for Dementia
Infection Awareness in Dementia Care
Medication Compliance for Dementia
Music Therapy for Dementia
Nutrition for Dementia
Placement for Dementia
Sundowning Management for Dementia

Connect with Peter On:

Website: https://compassioncrossing.info/